SO-BJO-236

Praise for Freedom From Disease

"Some of the most common health concerns we face today—diabetes, depression, fatigue, obesity and memory loss may be a consequence of insulin resistance. The authors clearly present the research that supports this assertion and the steps each and everyone of us must take to achieve a healthy life"

—Dr. Robert Goldman, MD, PhD, DO, FAASP, chairman of A4M International

"*Freedom from Disease* clearly and eloquently opens the eyes of its readers to the inherent risks and maladies lurking when the human machine is taken for granted and offers solutions to keep the most efficient machine known, the human body, well tuned."

—Dr. Robert Gotlin, Director of Orthopedic and Sports Rehabilitation at Beth Israel Medical Center and orthopedic consultant to the New York Knicks, Yankees, Liberty, and New Jersey Nets

"[The authors] have written an important and enjoyable book that should be of great interest to all. Particularly in the area of cardiovascular disease which is responsible for the most deaths in the US even exceeding cancer, they lay out the compelling interrelationship between insulin resistance and inflammation of the arterial wall leading to heart attack and ultimately to heart failure. The most important contribution of this book however is its "call to arms" and how individuals can influence their own health destiny by discipline in what they eat and how they exercise to prevent chronic disease."

—Dr. John C. Burnett, Jr., MD, Marriott Family Professor of Cardiovascular Research, Mayo Clinic

"The authors clearly document the current epidemic of obesity and the alarming increases in a number of diseases ranging from diabetes, heart disease, Alzheimer's and endocrine and immune pathologies, all due to the excess of sugar in western diets."

—Dr. Allan Goldstein, PhD, Chairman of Chemistry and Molecular Biology at George Washington University

Freedom

from

Disease

The Breakthrough Approach to Preventing Cancer, Heart Disease,
Alzheimer's, and Depression by Controlling Insulin and Inflammation

Peter M. Kash, EdD
Linda Friedland, MD
Jay Lombard, DO

DIVERSIONBOOKS

Diversion Books
A Division of Diversion Publishing Corp.
443 Park Avenue South, Suite 1008
New York, New York 10016
www.DiversionBooks.com

Copyright © 2008, 2017 by Dr. Peter M. Kash, Dr. Linda Friedland, and Dr. Jay Lombard
All rights reserved, including the right to reproduce this book or portions thereof in any form whatsoever.

For more information, email info@diversionbooks.com

First Diversion Books edition March 2017.
Print ISBN: 978-1-63576-113-9
eBook ISBN: 978-1-63576-112-2

Contents

We Stand on the Precipice

Our society's emphasis upon treating disease, as opposed to keeping people well, has just about run its course. In the relatively near future, our medical system, along with wide swaths of the American economy, will either be bankrupt or on the road to recovery. That's the crucial fork in the road that we will face in the twenty-first century. If the medical system goes bankrupt, our society will face widespread chaos. If we learn from our mistakes, we will evolve into a more sustainable, healthier culture. Individually, each of us will enjoy well-being—and all that that means— along with greater freedom from pharmaceutical drugs and avoidable medical procedures. Collectively, our society will be more creative and thus better able to direct our considerable resources toward other problems we currently face. As with every species, there are times when the conditions demand an evolutionary leap. Humanity now faces one of those times.

Essentially, our challenge is to change behaviors that have become a threat to our health and our ability to deliver medical services to all our people. The foods most of us are eating today and our lack of physical activity are poisoning our bodies and altering the way our central nervous systems function, thus causing a wide array of physical and mental disorders, as well as premature death.

As a professor and vice chair of surgery at New York Presbyterian-Columbia University Hospital, I see the effects of these behaviors every day in my medical practice and in the operating room. The sludge-filled coronary arteries, diseased gallbladders, fatty livers, hypertension-scarred kidneys, and cancerous tumors are just some of the consequences of our toxic lifestyle. Unbeknownst to most of us, so too are many of the mood and brain disorders that so many of us suffer from today.

Our health care system addresses the multiple epidemics we face by treating illness after it arises, rather than addressing the causes of disease at their source. Not surprisingly, medicine cannot keep pace with the rising rates of illness because we are treating people at the wrong end of the problem.

A great many of the diseases we face today arise from our inability to manage our weight, with more than two-thirds of Americans overweight, and more than a third obese. During the 1980s, little more than a third of Americans were overweight and only 15% were obese.

Similar disease patterns are emerging around the world. The World Health Organization has stated that more than 1 billion people worldwide are overweight and that about 300 million are now obese. Almost unbelievably, those who are overweight now outnumber those who are undernourished (there are now about 600 million hungry people worldwide).

The problem with overweight and obesity is that they have a domino effect on our biology. We don't just get fat. Overweight changes our internal chemistry so that the basic commands that are passed between cells, and within them, are dramatically altered. Soon this misinformation causes genes to malfunction, which in turn causes an array of illnesses, including diabetes, high blood pressure, heart disease, mood disorders, Alzheimer's disease, and many common cancers.

Obesity's partner in crime, diabetes, is now a worldwide epidemic. There are more than 29 million diabetics in the US today. By 2025, that number will likely double. By the year 2050, the number of people worldwide with diabetes will reach 250 million unless something is done to stop this raging epidemic. As with overweight, diabetes causes the widespread breakdown of health, raising the risk of infection, gangrene, amputation, blindness, kidney disorders, and heart attack.

In the past, illnesses such as diabetes and heart disease were considered diseases of old age, but all of that is changing. Today, we are seeing an ever-increasing number of children who are overweight, diabetic, and suffering from the early stages of heart disease—all ominous signs for our future.

Needless to say, treating these illnesses costs inconceivable sums of money. Today, annual health care costs in the

US hover at about two trillion dollars, two and one-half times what they were in 1990, and seven times what they were in 1980. The vast majority of this money is being spent on catastrophic care, especially the medical treatment received at the end of life. Half of the total health care bill for treating the average American over the course of his or her lifetime will be spent during that person's final eight years of life. If things continue as they are, the emergence of the baby boomers into old age—along with the multiple epidemics they'll suffer from—will crush our health care system. Unless something is done to improve our overall health, our society may be forced to limit medical care in order to curtail costs. Eventually, many will be shut out of the health care system, leaving increasing numbers of us sick and untreated. Such a reality would have a catastrophic effect on our society.

Turning things around

The question is: What can we do about it? Peter Kash, Linda Friedland and Jay Lombard have provided a penetrating analysis of what's going wrong in the human body, and what we all can do to restore our health. As their insightful book shows, overweight, diabetes, heart disease, Alzheimer's, many mood disorders, and common forms of cancer all seem to stem from the same underlying root causes. The causes are insulin resistance and inflammation.

Insulin, a hormone produced by the body that allows blood sugar to enter cells and be utilized as fuel, is a key regulator that determines health and illness for most of us today. When we eat foods that drive insulin levels up, and keep them elevated, cellular function is altered and cells behave in aberrant ways, thus forming the basis for many of the diseases we face today.

How does it do it? By changing the communication that flows between cells.

One of the great insights the authors of this book make clear is cells talk to each other. In this way, they maintain order throughout the system. Health is a consequence of that order. When cellular communication occurs normally, the body functions as it was designed to—flawlessly.

One of the key regulators of cellular communication is insulin. In decades past, we doctors used to think that this hormone's sole job was to regulate the flow of energy into cells. And while this is, in fact, one of insulin's principle functions, we now know that it does a great deal more than simply act as a gatekeeper for energy. Insulin, it turns out, dramatically affects the flow of information that takes place within cells, as well as between them, and thus regulates how cells behave. When insulin levels are healthy and balanced, cells function with awesome precision. The result for each of us is good health. But when insulin levels become elevated, and remain high over time, cellular communication breaks down. Cells behave in strange and disorderly ways, thus forming the basis for the epidemics we see today.

The good news is that all of us can control our insulin levels by virtue of controlling the nutrients we consume, and the amount of physical activity in which we engage each day. That means that we can, to a great extent, control how our cells function and, by extension, determine for ourselves whether or not we experience good health.

As I frequently tell my patients, as well as the people who tune in to my television show, medicine can do a great deal to help you defeat disease and restore your health. But the truth is, you can do more than we doctors can.

Peter Kash, Linda Friedland and Jay Lombard's book shows how you can protect yourself from serious illness, and, in many cases, restore your health if you are already ill. By controlling the foods you eat, the nutrient levels in your body, and the amount of exercise you engage in, you can regulate this essential hormone, reduce inflammation, and in the process give yourself the gift of good health.

Mehmet Oz, MD

CHAPTER 1

Insulin: A Key to Health and Illness

Scientists have long dreamed of the day when they would discover that single agent within the human body that causes many of the illnesses that afflict and kill us. With such knowledge, we could transform the source of disease, restore the body's biochemical balance, and thus prevent heart disease, many cancers, diabetes, and obesity—we might even prevent serious degenerative brain disorders, such as Alzheimer's and Parkinson's, as well as conditions that afflict children, including attention deficit hyperactivity disorder (ADHD). Such knowledge could one day form the basis for effective treatments for these conditions, as well.

The good news is that much of this is now within your

personal control. That remarkable discovery may have already been made. Not only have we identified one of the underlying sources of many serious illnesses, we are also learning how to manipulate it successfully to prevent and treat many of the diseases just named. That singular, pivotal factor, central in many of today's disorders, is insulin, the hormone produced by the pancreas that allows blood sugar to enter cells.

Not just sugar

Most people know that insulin is directly involved in the creation of diabetes, an illness that now afflicts some 30 million Americans and 415 million globally including an ever-growing number of children and young adults. One in two adults with diabetes (46%) is undiagnosed. But the ill effects of insulin go far beyond diabetes. Insulin, scientists have found, is one of the body's master chemicals, regulating an enormous number of other biological functions downstream.

When maintained at balanced levels, insulin ensures the steady flow of energy to your cells. It helps create a healthy body weight, supports the health of your heart and circulatory system, and protects you from many common cancers. It also maintains your emotional health and the clarity of your mind and memory.

When it is elevated, and remains chronically high, insulin can act like a diabolical computer programmer, rewriting your cellular command codes and wreaking havoc throughout the body. Far from being just a catalyst for diabetes, elevated insulin plays a central role in virtually every major illness we face today, including overweight, obesity, heart disease, cancer, and Alzheimer's disease. It may also have some role in the creation of attention deficit hyperactivity disorder, mood imbalances, and mental illness.

Every cell needs energy

This simple hormone has such a widespread effect on health because every biological act requires energy. Insulin is needed if cells are to use that energy, which means insulin is involved in all human functions. The sheer ubiquity of the hormone gives it entrée into virtually every nook and cranny, every cell, organ, and system of your body. We all remember tenth grade biology, trying to understand the connection between mitochondria, energy, and ATP. This has a direct connection to insulin resistance and type 2 diabetes. Consequently, insulin can be a help or a hindrance in everything the body does.

How food works

To a great extent, we can control our insulin levels by virtue of the kinds of foods we eat, the quantity of calories we consume, how much we exercise, and how well we cope with stress.

Processed foods, such as bagels, muffins, pastries, candy, and soda, for example, are all rich in calories. They are also packed with the kinds of simple carbohydrates— otherwise known as simple sugars—that drive insulin levels through the roof. Foods high in fat are also rich in calories and can also contribute to high insulin levels. By keeping insulin levels elevated, these foods *may* contribute to all the degenerative illnesses that afflict most of us today.

On the other hand, unprocessed foods—cooked whole grains, fresh vegetables, beans, and fruit—and many low fat animal products are low in calories and keep insulin levels stable. This is one of the major reasons why these foods are associated with good health and longer life.

Exercise lowers insulin; stress drives it up

Exercise, even a simple walk around the block, lowers insulin levels and makes cells more sensitive to the insulin that's in the blood. That means that the body utilizes insulin more efficiently—in other words, a little goes a long way.

In addition, stress drives up insulin levels and chronic stress keeps insulin levels high. This is one of the ways stress contributes to a variety of major illnesses and premature death—it drives insulin levels up.

Only recently did researchers become aware of insulin's central role in health. But already, scientists have developed new pharmaceutical agents that protect us against the destructive chemical cascade that insulin triggers within our cells.

In fact, the understanding of insulin's role in health and illness is revolutionizing health care. New forms of treatment offer hope even for those of us who already suffer from one of the many diseases brought about by chronically high insulin levels.

A tiny flame

One of the most baffling mysteries of disease is how it arises. What conditions allow a tiny and dangerous flame within us to become a blazing threat to our lives? Is it true that the body, for no discernible reason, suddenly breaks down, malfunctions, and sets loose a disease process? Or is it possible that an array of poisons—many of which we control—combine to target a single weak link within us, a link that, when it breaks down, sets off a terrible chain reaction?

For millions of us today, that is precisely what happens. That vulnerable link within us may be due to pathways of insulin or other important hormones and chemicals.

Computer programmer

Groups of researchers have been working for some time on insulin's relationship to specific illnesses such as heart disease and cancer. Each of the groups focused on their own area of expertise. Only recently has insulin been confirmed as a possible common trigger in virtually all serious illnesses.

Insulin is a kind of computer programmer, determining where signals are sent within the human body. Depending on the skill of that programmer, we can experience good health, vitality, and efficient brain function, or we can suffer weight increases, internal chaos, an endless variety of negative health states.

The growing awareness of insulin's pivotal role in health is changing the way we treat disease, and bringing forth a new model for health and illness.

Scientists now realize that the human body is the most elaborate and complex array of information highways.

A living supercomputer

Your body can be seen as a living, breathing supercomputer. The health of that supercomputer depends on its ability to send life-sustaining information from one cell to another. This is no different from sending a text or WhatsApp. That same information must also be transferred to specific sites within cells so that cells function properly.

Illness arises when disruptive or chaotic commands are sent to cells, which in turn causes them to behave in self-destructive ways. (No different from some of our teenagers' behaviors!)

In short, proper functioning of the body depends on the information being sent throughout the system.

All of which brings us back to that central pancreatic hormone that we know as insulin. This chemical substance is, in fact, one of the body's central messengers, telling cells to perform an array of essential tasks.

Cells need sugar

The first job of insulin is instructing cells to absorb blood sugar, also known as glucose, which is the body's primary fuel. Cells need glucose to perform their tasks; in essence, they need it to survive. Without blood sugar, cells die.

At the same time, insulin also triggers a series of internal signals within the cells, some of which eventually make their way to genes, which in turn direct the cell to perform some kind of task.

Here comes the problem. When insulin levels become elevated—and remain high—bad signals get passed to cells and sometimes to your genetic coding which, once disrupted, can possibly cause a number of serious diseases. The important point to remember for now is that insulin regulates much of the information that gets inside your cells.

Disorders such as obesity, diabetes, heart disease, cancer, and brain and nervous system disorders appear to be quite different from each other. But let us imagine that each of these illnesses is a specific byproduct, a kind of terrible fruit that springs from the same tree. That tree is called *insulin resistance*.

Insulin resistance

Like any machine, the body needs only a limited amount of fuel to run properly. But unlike other machines, excess fuel is dangerous to the human body. So the body does everything it can to push this excess fuel into storage, and this is the main job of insulin. The way it can cause serious harm is this: As the sugar levels rise, the body experiences dramatic shifts in fluid levels, increasing the risk of edema throughout the system, including in the brain. Brain swelling can lead to coma and death. At the same time, elevations in blood sugar can cause electrolyte levels to drop. Electrolytes are the minerals in cells that facilitate the flow of electrical signals throughout the system. As electrolyte levels fall, organs begin to malfunction. Among the most vulnerable is the heart, which can go into arrhythmia and fail.

In order to avoid that fate, the body employs a number of strategies, one of which is to burn off as much of the excess fuel as it can. When there is too much sugar in your blood, the brain signals the pancreas to produce more insulin, and insulin forces the excess sugar into cells so that it can be burned as energy. Unfortunately, if the cells are already filled to capacity with sugar and they don't want any more fuel, they close their doors and become resistant to the additional glucose. The excess blood sugar remains, but if it's not taken care of you will die. So, doing what it must, the body produces even more insulin, which can then force the excess sugar into cells. Additional insulin can overcome the cell's resistance, but as more and more sugar floods the bloodstream, cells become even more resistant. (This is why doctors and dieticians tell us not to reach for that extra bagel at midnight while watching reruns of *How I Met Your Mother*.)

Overstimulated

When cells are persistently overstimulated by a particular signal—in this case insulin—they eventually become insensitive to that signal. In effect, they become resistant to it. High levels of glucose and insulin in the blood cause the insulin receptors on cells to become insensitive to insulin signaling. That's especially the case when the cell is already filled to capacity with glucose.

Insulin resistance is essentially a condition in which

cells are rejecting the fuel they need to not only function efficiently but to live. Without fuel, cells die, so the organs they compose (heart, kidneys, etc.) become heavily scarred with dead cells and tissues and then lose their functional capacities.

Becoming fat

Worldwide obesity and overweight has doubled. In 2017, according to WHO, 1.9 billion are overweight and 600 million are obese. In the US alone, 17% of children are obese. As cells turn glucose and insulin away, more of both fill the bloodstream. The body is forced to convert the excess glucose into fat, which accumulates in the blood and throughout our bodies. Some of that fat is stored on the waistline, buttocks, thighs, shoulders, and back, causing excess weight gain. Even more fat forms around the heart and other organs, forcing them to have to work harder to get the job done. Meanwhile, globules of fat infiltrate the blood, cutting off the oxygen supply to cells and organs and possibly causing them to suffocate.

Insulin resistance may also lead to higher levels of inflammation (see chapter 2) which further exacerbates the entire disease process.

The accumulating fat on our bodies coupled with high insulin levels, causes your fatty tissues to produce chemicals that may also change the way the cells in your brain function, altering brain chemistry and creating biochemical changes that may lead to memory loss and dementia.

Elevated insulin levels create a domino effect that can

lead to devastating damage in many systems and organs in the body, including signaling the formation of cancer cells.

Breaking the destructive cycle

Now that insulin has been implicated in many health problems, scientists are investigating how they can intercept the bad commands initiated by insulin and insert new information that would cause the cell to react properly. In fact, new drugs are now being developed to do exactly that in many areas of health care. In the meantime, there is much each of us can do to protect ourselves and those we love, even without our doctor's help.

Controlling insulin is important not only from the standpoint of prevention, but also for those who are already ill. Lowering insulin levels can have a dramatic and restorative effect on health, and in many cases, help people overcome life-threatening illnesses. We can prevent disease, restore our health, and also bring our health care costs down.

But in order to do all of that, we must better understand the enormous role insulin plays in the complex and delicate communication that takes place within our bodies.

Insulin signaling is involved in the multiple epidemics we face today, including overweight, obesity, heart disease, and certain cancers, and may possibly also play some role in hyperactive and attention deficit disorders in children, and an explosion of neurological diseases, including Alzheimer's. On the face of it, all of these illnesses look distinctly different from one another. But as scientists investigate their deeper origins, they are discovering that many illnesses may spring from the same underlying common pathways, biological systems, and overlapping mechanisms of disease such as insulin resistance, inflammation, and mitochondrial dysfunction.

We need to break this cycle and lead by example. Take a walk with your spouse and kids instead of watching an extra hour of bad news! Make excellent choices about what food you eat and what you feed your children. Ensure you have strategies in place such as yoga, martial arts, meditation, or golf to defuse your stress. Although you may have zero control over the happenings in this crazy world, you can have an enormous impact on your own health and the well-being of your family!

CHAPTER 2

———

Pathways to Disease: New Thinking

Systems biology

There's a new term used in health, science, research, and medicine. "Systems biology" is the study of systems of biological components, which may be molecules, cells, organisms, or entire species. Living systems are dynamic and complex, and their behavior may be hard to predict from the properties of individual parts.

The definition and explanation directly from the Institute for Systems Biology, Seattle, leading experts in the function and behavior of every organ in the human body, is that "[systems biology] is a holistic approach to deciphering the complexity of biological systems that starts from the understanding that the networks that form the whole of living organisms are more than the sum of their parts. It is collaborative, integrating many scientific disciplines—biology, computer science, engineering, bioinformatics, physics and others—to predict how these systems change over time and under varying conditions, and to develop solutions to the world's most pressing health issues."

Old medical model

Up until the recent past, most illnesses were seen as the result of a general destruction of the body, usually caused by an array of environmental poisons or a pathogen, such as a bacteria or virus. No common cause of disease could be identified, nor was there any unified theory concerning health and illness. Rather, scientists and doctors saw various disease states as individual conditions, most of which were unrelated to each other. Under the old medical model, doctors and pharmaceutical companies were restricted to treating the symptoms of disease, rather than the underlying cause of it. Not only has our lack of understanding of the root causes of illness limited our ability to offer more effective treatments, but it has also kept us from creating new programs for prevention.

We now know this not to be true. Our bodies are made up of countless interdependent networks and overlapping mechanisms of disease. There are several common pathways working together.

New medical model: integrated networks

On a biological level, our bodies are made up of integrated networks that communicate on multiple levels. Our genes, DNA, molecules, and the cells that make up our organs are all interacting through a network of networks now generally called *systems biology.*

"Systems biology is based on the understanding that the whole is greater than the sum of the parts," explains Dr. Leroy Hood, the president and cofounder of the Institute for Systems Biology. Systems biology has been responsible for some of the most important developments in the science of human health. It is a totally holistic approach to unraveling the complexity of human structure and function.

"The knee bone is connected to the thigh bone"

"It is no longer enough to understand only one part of a system when studying the complexity of biology and how our bodies stay healthy or break down. It used to be as simple as 'the knee bone connected to the thigh bone.' Now scientists use systems biology approaches to understand the big picture of how all the pieces interact in an organism by putting its pieces together. It's in stark contrast to decades of reductionist biology, which involves taking the pieces apart," explains Dr. Hood.

Cells, tissues, organs, and body systems

Our body is an extremely complex system made up of many parts, each performing specific functions. A cell (of which there are trillions in the body) is made up of organelles. These organelles interact to maintain a healthy cell and also send signals to neighboring cells. Hundreds of thousands of *cells* make up a multicellular system called *tissue*. Examples of tissues are muscle, epithelial tissue (such as skin) and connective tissue. A group of different tissues makes up an *organ*, for example our liver, kidney, or heart. Two or more organs work together to form a *system*, such as the nervous system or cardiovascular system. These organ systems all interact with each other to maintain healthy functioning.

One cell: an entire blueprint for life

Within each cell are several vital subcellular structures such as the mitochondria (cell *battery*) filled with energy, lysosomes containing enzymes and proteins, and the nucleus within which resides DNA containing our genetic material. The magnificent complexity of how cells actually "think," "communicate," and "respond" to messages are explained in great detail in the next chapter. An intriguing concept is that each cell in a group of supposedly identical cells is a distinct entity. "There is no 'average cell' even within a population of cells of the very same cell type," explains Dr. Hood. Just as individual people within a population group may fall into specific subgroups, there are also discrete cell subtypes in a cell population. These cell subtypes perform different functions and form a network, much like a social network in human populations. The advanced scientific study of systems biology requires us to view tissues and organs as dynamic populations of integrated cells and not as an amorphous mass.

What are proteomics & genomics?

Proteomics is the large-scale study of proteins and their structures and functions. Proteins are the molecules that make life happen. They are the machinery that turn food into cell energy, make cells move, and most importantly they are the mini computers that literally read the DNA and make more proteins. If DNA is the blueprint for life, then proteins are the bricks. They are simply chains of amino acids. The specific type and order of the amino acids in a protein will change its shape and determine its specific function.

The term "proteomics" was created in the 1990s to make an analogy with genomics—the study of the genome. Just as genomics is the study of the entire set of genes found in living things, the proteome is the entire set of proteins.

The genome: an instruction manual

The genome, a combination of the words "gene" and "chromosome," is the complete set of hereditary instructions in each cell of every living thing that is needed by the organism for its development and functioning. It is similar to an instruction manual on how cells work. So if we use the book metaphor, our genome is the book, our chromosomes are the chapters of the book, the genes are the sentences, and the DNA the letters forming words and sentences. To continue the metaphor, a genetic mutation could best be explained as a typographical error and a genetic variation as a spelling variation. The information needed to build every protein in an organism is contained in the DNA. The genes in DNA are translated into these proteins, simply strings of amino acids that fold into three-dimensional structures. Different proteins are produced in different amounts, at different times, and with different functions. For example, a cell in your ear and a cell in your gut may contain identical DNA but completely different subsets of proteins, which give each its special function.

Epigenetics

Epigenetics is the fascinating science within genetics that explains how we might have some control even over our genes. In simplified terms, epigenetics is the study of biological mechanisms that switch genes on and off. Certain circumstances in life can cause genes to be turned off (becoming dormant) or turned on (becoming active). What we eat, what environment we find ourselves in, how we sleep, what type of exercise we do—all of these can eventually cause chemical changes to turn certain genes on or off over time. With more than 20,000 genes, what will be the result of different combinations of genes being turned on or off? The possible variations are enormous! But if we could map every single cause and effect of the different combinations, and if we could reverse the gene's state to keep the good while eliminating the bad…then we could theoretically cure cancer, slow aging, stop obesity, and so much more.

We have significant power through our mental state. There is a remarkable connection between our brains and our bodies. Our thoughts, emotions, and attitudes are converted into chemicals that communicate directly with our metabolism, immunity, our cells, and even our genes. Right down to the genetic level, you do in fact have personal influence.

"How wonderful that the billions of cells in our bodies each have their own personalities," explains Pulitzer Prize–winning author of *Emperor of all Maladies* and professor of medicine at Columbia University Dr. Siddhartha Mukherjee.

There are several common overlapping pathways that contribute to damage and destruction, aging and illness. Despite the numerous mutations and mechanisms that are way beyond our control, there is much in systems biology within our power to influence and change. A basic understanding of these somewhat complicated pathways provides crystalline clarity about the importance of our lifestyle choices.

Freedom from disease will highlight the interconnected and overlapping pathways of inflammation, insulin resistance and mitochondrial dysfunction throughout all aspects of this book.

All disease begins in the gut?

Hippocrates once said that "all diseases begin in the gut." This seemed a preposterous suggestion up until fairly recently. We have discovered that the gut is so much more than a digestive organ. It is one of the fundamental components of immunity, and it is vital to our metabolism, but most fascinating is that it may in fact be a second brain!

So much more than simple bugs!

At least 100 trillion bacteria live in and on your body. Some are present on the surface of the skin and inside the mouth, nose, and urogenital tract—but most live within your gut. The gut flora is the complex community of microorganisms that live in our digestive tracts. The presence of these bacteria in our gut is fundamental to most aspects of our health.

What do the gut microbes do?

The intestinal flora helps to detox the toxins and carcinogens that come through our digestive tract. They stimulate the digestive process and aid the absorption of nutrients. They produce vital life-supporting vitamins B and K. They help regulate the growth of the gut cells and keep them healthy. These 100 trillion microbes in the human gut amazingly have a direct effect on our neurological functions, our moods, and possibly our mental health. They mostly train the immune system to recognize and fight harmful bacteria. This helps protect the body from disease.

Are there bad gut microbes?

Just as, in your garden, weeds compete for space and nutrients and "choke out" healthy plants, so "bad" bacteria behave the same way in your intestines, potentially threatening your health. In a healthy gut flora, the effects of the good bacteria outweigh the effects of harmful sorts.

How to keep the balance

The composition of human gut flora changes over time, when the diet changes, and as overall health changes. An unhealthy diet, excess stress, various illnesses, travel, changes in water composition, and even just getting older can diminish your good gut microbes. Attempt to keep the balance with optimal nutrition, good food hygiene, and being careful what you eat and drink when you travel.

The easiest way to keep your good microbes alive and thriving is by eating food enriched with powerful probiotics such as best-quality yogurt with live cultures of probiotics. You may remember the famous Dannon Yogurt commercial. Did you rush out and buy the blueberry flavor after watching this hilarious commercial, ranked in top 100 of all time? The 89-year-old Russian, with his ancient 110-year-old mother by his side, consumes two cups of yogurt followed by the comment, "[T]hat pleased his mother very much." Another way to increase your intake of good bacteria is through eating naturally fermented food like sauerkraut, kimchi, or kombucha.

Different microbes in the obese vs. lean

Gut microbiota have a powerful effect of insulin resistance. In the publication *Nutrients* March 2013, "The role of gut microbiota on insulin resistance" by Caricelli and Saad demonstrated that the bacterial load as well as the specific types of bacteria in obese individuals differs from a lean person. There was an increase in Firmicutes and Actinobacteria but a decrease in Bacteroidetes in the overweight group. These differences led to increased inflammation pathways, which then led to alterations in insulin. Metabolic syndrome and obesity may change the environment in the gut so that different bacteria thrives or is subdued, affecting the overall health of a patient.

What is the brain-gut axis?

The *gut-brain axis* is the biochemical signaling that takes place between the gastrointestinal (GI) tract and the central nervous system. That term has been expanded to include the role of the gut flora in the interplay; the term "microbiome-gut-brain axis" is sometimes used to describe this system. As strange as it sounds, endotoxins created by bacterial byproducts disrupt not only the gut but also its interactions with the brain. Psychological stress has long been anecdotally reported to increase disease activity in inflammatory bowel disease (IBD), and recent well-designed studies have confirmed that. Stress is a huge trigger of microbial imbalances, which can lead to inflammation and possible ill health. Mawdsley and Rampton in the publication of *Gut* in October 2005 demonstrated how chronic-stress-induced alterations in gastrointestinal function and can lead to IBS (Irritable Bowel Syndrome) by stimulating the pituitary gland to release the hormones that ultimately lead to secretion of cortisol, which has potent effects. Chronic stress leads to other potential health issues such as gastroesophageal reflux disease and gastric or duodenal ulcers. It also, may affect sleep and eating patterns.

The second brain?

The gut's nervous system is called the enteric nervous system and is one of the main divisions of the main nervous system, i.e. the brain and spinal cord. It consists of a mesh-like system of brain cells (neurons) that govern the function of the gastrointestinal tract. It has been described as a "second brain" for several reasons, most importantly because the enteric nervous system can actually operate autonomously. So you could say the gut is thinking and feeling on its own, independent of the brain!

Anxiety? Autism? Energy? Gut bacteria link?

Dr. Sarkis Mazmanian of Californian Institute of Technology postulates in the Journal *Cell* (December 2013) that there may be some correlation of low levels of *Bacteroides Fragilis* in children with autism. Dr. Stephen Collins from McMaster University in Ontario found that the increased intake of *Lactobacillus* and *Bifidobacterium* reduces anxiety in mice. A new study (2016) in the Journal *Nutrition in Clinical Practice* shows that microorganisms in the human gastrointestinal tract form an intricate, living fabric of natural controls affecting body weight and, especially, energy.

Inflammation

What is usually a totally normal, short-lived essential response to an invading virus or bacteria or injury can become a damaging process when it occurs unabated for long periods of time.

Most of us suffer from some degree of chronic inflammation, caused by a variety of factors that may seriously undermine our health and age us prematurely. Most of the time we are totally unaware of this pathway as this inflammation is low grade. Chronic inflammation generates a constant supply of damaging substances that overwhelm our defenses and cause damage. With time this common pathway may cause diseases of every description.

Resulting from an "inflammatory cascade" that continues unabated for decades, common chronic conditions may manifest, such as arthritis, autoimmune diseases, diabetes, gastrointestinal conditions, heart disease and Alzheimer's.

What is inflammation?

Inflammation is the body's normal response to any irritation, infection, or injury. For the most part it is a natural and healthy bodily process.

If you cut your finger, the body immediately begins an inflammatory process that neutralizes harmful microorganisms, helps to repair the wound, and cleans up the debris resulting from the injury. *Inflammation is beneficial when needed in an acute situation, but it is disastrous when chronic.*

The signs of normal inflammation

The signs of normal inflammation—pain, heat, swelling and redness—are the first indications that your immune system has kicked into action.

When an injury or invasion of organism occurs, your

body releases white blood cells into the blood and into the affected site to fight off and protect your body from these foreign substances. The different specialized white cells called neutrophils and macrophages release chemicals. These chemicals increase blood flow, resulting in redness and heat in the specific area. They also cause a leakage of fluid into the tissues, which causes swelling and may stimulate nerve endings, causing pain.

Acute inflammation that occurs in the body when needed and recedes immediately thereafter signifies a well-balanced immune system. But when the signs and symptoms of inflammation don't fade away, it's a signal that the immune system switch remains stuck at "on." Your immune system remains on high alert—even when you aren't in imminent danger—and the inflammation continues unabated. The system just won't shut off.

Inflammation: a major cause of bodily damage

Inflammation—a system designed to protect the body from harm—when unabated becomes a serious cause of bodily damage. It is thought to be at the core of a vast number of chronic illnesses. It is one of the most significant and common pathways in the development of disease. Inflammation, insulin resistance, and mitochondrial dysfunction are probably the three most common pathways towards illness and bodily damage.

Heart attack, heart disease, and stroke (the commonest causes of death in developed nations) are due to reduced blood flow through narrowed and damaged blood vessels.

Up until fairly recently this was thought to be primarily due to the fatty plaques that develop in the lining of these arteries. The real cause of damage is the *inflammation* in these vessels concurrent with the fatty deposits. Damage within the brain leading to Alzheimer's and other forms of dementia is due to the development of brain plaques. These plaques have their origin in inflammatory tissue.

Tests for inflammation?

Currently there is no definitive test for inflammation. The best measure available in conventional medicine is a blood test called CRP, C-reactive protein, which is a nonspecific marker of inflammation. Testing for a ratio of lipid proteins called Apolipoprotein B and Apolipoprotein A1 is also being used through some medical centers.

What causes chronic inflammation?

Inflammation is one of the common denominators of disease. Almost every very chronic disease has an element of inflammatory disease. Learning how to possibly prevent and reverse inflammation may be a key in the prevention and possible reversal of disease processes, as well as slowing the aging process and keeping us healthy.

There are numerous possible causes of chronic inflammation.

1. Environmental causes. Pesticides, pollution, and heavy metals such as lead and mercury are just some of the substances in our environment that our bodies must detoxify. Cleaning products, plastics, adhesives, air fresheners, latex, and glues are some of the vast array of other chemicals we are exposed to every day. Many of us work in sealed office buildings with recirculated air that only increases our exposure. Many of these toxins are in our drinking water and our food. A large proportion of these chemicals are fat-soluble, meaning they are stored in fat and accumulate in our bodies, where they may eventually reach toxic levels. There is some preliminary data that demonstrates that many of these environmental factors may be playing havoc with our immune systems and contributing to inflammation throughout the body. Some people are naturally better detoxifiers and can withstand more exposure before they experience any damage.

2. Hormonal causes. Hormones work on so many levels, several of which we don't fully understand yet. It is difficult to identify the exact process but we do know that hormones affect inflammation. Changing levels of estrogen, progesterone, and testosterone may have a role to play in age-related inflammation. In women it is thought that prior to menopause the balance of hormones has a calming effect on inflammation, whereas the symptoms of chronic inflammation often become more apparent during and after menopause. Although we don't understand all the pathways, it appears that a decrease in estrogen corresponds with a rise in the cytokines called interleukin-1 and interleukin-6. The hormonal changes leading up to menopause also contribute to weight gain. And there is clear evidence that extra fat cells, especially around the midriff region of the body, add to systemic inflammation by creating extra cytokines.

3. Inflammation originating from the gut. Some researched data reveals that general inflammation throughout the body may originate in the GI tract. Heartburn and acid reflux are early signs of an inflamed digestive tract. Our digestive tract is a powerful component of the body's immune system. It is designed to eliminate viruses and bacteria acquired through our food before they reach the rest of our body. We give our digestive systems plenty of work to do. Our diet, high in processed, refined, and convenience food, is overwhelming our metabolic pathways (see "insulin resistance" below) and our digestive tract. This, too much sugar, high levels of common allergens, and insufficient probiotics (good bacteria), are some of the supposed triggers of inflammation.

4. Foods that cause inflammation. Our Western diet is generally proinflammatory. It is rich in proinflammatory compounds, while lacking antioxidants and other nutrients that help to prevent and control inflammation.

- *Sugar and refined carbs.* For most people, high-carbohydrate diets are inflammatory. Refined foods with a high glycemic index and sugar in particular spike up insulin levels, exacerbating inflammation.

  Unaware of this, the average American consumes more than 160 pounds of sugar and 200 pounds of white flour per year. Sugar and white flour increase blood sugar levels, and even a modest increase generates proinflammatory chemicals.

The mechanism is a complicated interplay of various hormones, enzymes and acids. Specific hormones called eicosanoids, located inside our cells, act as either pro- or anti-inflammatory compounds depending on their type. When insulin levels are high, these eicosanoids become imbalanced and stimulate more inflammation.

- *Acidity* is another problem. Most Americans eat an acidic diet of too much salt, sugar, white flour, dairy, meat, and cola drinks. Many experts consider high acidity to be one of the major causes of chronic inflammation.

- *Omega fats imbalance.* The fats and oils in the American diet are inflammatory because they contain excessive omega-6 fatty acids. Omega-6 fatty acids are proinflammatory, while omega-3s are anti-inflammatory. Historically, humans consumed roughly equal amounts of these oils, achieving a balance. Today, we consume 20 to 30 times as much omega-6 as omega-3. The modern processed-food industry fills our stores with proinflammatory oils, including corn, sunflower, soy, canola, and peanut oils. Grain-fed beef, poultry, and farmed fish also contain excessive omega-6. These imbalances create a huge excess of pro-inflammatory chemicals in our diet. Hence the need to eat more fatty fish, flax seed, or take an omega 3 supplement.

- *Hydrogenated oils* are also proinflammatory. Trans fats, which are found in margarine and most processed foods, are good fats that have been rendered toxic through hydrogenation. This is done in order to make liquid oils solid at room temperature. TFAs (trans fatty acids) are a potent stimulus for inflammation throughout the body. These oils find their way into most processed products, including candy, baked goods, margarine, breakfast cereal, and peanut butter. The trans fatty acids contained in hydrogenated oils inhibit the activity of enzymes that make anti-inflammatory compounds, but not those that create proinflammatory ones; chronic inflammation is the result.

  They create renegade cells called free radicals that damage healthy cells and trigger this inflammation.

- *Food intolerance and allergy.* Some individuals may be intolerant of certain substances such as casein (found in milk) or gluten (found in wheat) which triggers the inflammatory cascade. There are those that are severely intolerant, such as sufferers of celiac disease.

- *Advanced glycation end products, or AGEs.* In addition, sugar and white flour cause inflammation and disease by forming AGEs. AGEs are produced when a protein reacts with sugar, resulting in damaged, cross-linked proteins. As the body tries to protect itself by breaking these AGEs apart, immune cells secrete large amounts of inflammatory chemicals. Many of the diseases that we think of as part of aging are actually caused by this process. Depending on where the AGEs occur, the result can be arthritis, heart disease, cataracts, memory loss, wrinkled skin, or diabetes complications, to name a few.

5. Psychological stress—cortisol and inflammation. Acute stress in the "fight or flight" response triggers the release of adrenaline and the stress hormone cortisol from your adrenal glands. When stress becomes chronic and sustained for long periods, large amounts of cortisol are circulating in your blood. Cortisol directly influences your insulin levels and metabolism. It also plays a role in chronic inflammation and your immune system. Coping with persistent stress takes a steady toll on your immune system, your adrenals, and your central nervous system. Your body reacts to stress in the same way whether it is biological or psychological. The more acute the threat feels, the more dramatic the response will be. Emotions and thoughts are very powerful and manifest themselves physically all the time with symptoms of inflammation. With all the other factors contributing to inflammation, stress is often overlooked—but it's really important.

6. Obesity and fat cells. Another promoter of chronic, systemic inflammation is fat cells. More than two out of three Americans are overweight, and fat cells, especially those that form around the abdomen, produce large amounts of inflammatory chemicals. This is a huge source of inflammation, and is the reason why overweight people may suffer much more disease and disability.

Why chronic inflammation is on the rise

Our bodies are not designed for the daily barrage of toxins, infectious agents, and stress. Although we have a highly effective immune system and can detoxify and withstand the onslaught of many different viral, bacterial, and toxic particles, much of our lifestyle today overwhelms this system. Whatever we breathe, eat, drink, and absorb has either a pro- or anti-inflammatory effect and most of the time the factors are skewed toward inflammation.

Well-documented research links mental and psychological stress, anxiety, and depression with the rise of inflammatory markers, such as CRP, signaling an increased risk for atherosclerosis and coronary heart disease (CHD).

Ways to combat chronic inflammation

Countering chronic inflammation takes a combination approach because it arises from a combination of causes. The good news is that much of it is in your control.

A diet high in a variety of fresh vegetables, fruits, nuts, and seeds is a powerful way to help calm the overwhelmingly powerful inflammatory processes occurring throughout the body. Although healing superfood is the first line of defense, there is a place for adding supplements and nutraceuticals to help ease bodily inflammation. The best nutrients include omega-3 fatty acids, vitamins

A, B complex (including folic acid, B6 and B12), C, D, and E, plus beta-carotene, CoQ10, curcumin, selenium, N-acetylcysteine, and lipoic acid.

Mitochondria: The Batteries of the Body

Mitochondria are specialized structures within every cell of the human body. They serve as batteries, powering various functions of the cell and the body as a whole.

Their main function is to generate energy in the form of a chemical molecule called ATP, which stands for adenosine triphosphate. They are the energy currency for all bodily functions, from muscle contraction to hormone production. When mitochondria fail, this results in a poor supply of ATP, so cells slow because they do not have the energy supply to function at a normal speed. This means that all bodily functions slow.

Mitochondria are recognized as major contributors to human health and disease.

Inherited verse acquired mitochondrial dysfunction

When mitochondrial dysfunction is inherited (of primary origin), it can be extremely dangerous and often fatal. This primary dysfunction results from mitochondrial DNA (mtDNA) mutations inherited from the infant's mother. Secondary (acquired) mitochondrial dysfunction may result from the influence of external mechanisms such as the environment, or pharmacologic toxins that can damage the mtDNA. Mitochondria are generally able to protect themselves from damage through various quality-control mechanisms. However, if these mechanisms are altered, mitochondrial dysfunction can lead to disease. Past research has predominantly focused on the role of mitochondrial dysfunction on disease pathology. However, some studies have investigated how mitochondrial dysfunction may be associated with the development of distressing symptoms such as fatigue, chronic pain, and depression. These investigations are still in their infancy.

Poor Stamina

The ATP energy pathway is a complicated metabolic process of what is called oxidative phosphorylation. The ATP is broken down to ADP (adenosine biphosphate) and back again to ATP. It is thought to recycle approximately every 10 seconds in a normal person—if this slows, then the cell slows, and so the person slows and clinically has poor stamina. The biological basis for poor stamina may indeed arise within mitochondria. (This mustn't be confused with serious inherited primary mitochondrial disease as discussed above.)

One can only go at the rate at which mitochondria can produce ATP. If mitochondria go slowly, stamina is poor.

At this stage much research is ongoing in the field of inherited mitochondrial dysfunction and for most infants born with severe inherited Mito disease, there is as yet no cure.

Secondary mitochondrial dysfunction is a totally different issue, where some insult to the body has occurred and the mitochondria are not functioning efficiently. There is no simple solution, but undoubtedly there are strategies that can help. Pace yourself—do not use up energy faster than your mitochondria can supply it. Get excellent sleep allowing your mitochondria to repair themselves as best as possible. Feed the mitochondria correctly, stabilizing blood sugar levels and avoiding as many toxins as possible, such as alcohol, tobacco, and household pesticides and chemicals. It is also important to try and address the underlying trigger with your healthcare provider, identifying any allergies, chronic infections, autoimmune conditions, liver detoxification problems, or digestive or hormonal problems.

CHAPTER 3

———

Cell Communication: Cells Talk to Each Other!

Cells communicate for health

It's a little hard for us to imagine that the chemicals passed between cells—including hormones, such as insulin—are actually loaded with information, but that's precisely the case. Molecular compounds, such as insulin, tell cells to behave in distinct ways. These chemicals direct the immune system to produce more natural killer cells, for example, or to attack a virus or bacteria within the system. These chemicals tell cells to reproduce, or to remain stable, or even to self-destruct. In fact, scientists have recently learned that health is the consequence of life-sustaining information being passed between cells, and then to specific targets within them. When that information reaches its intended destination, your cells, organs, and indeed, your entire body, function with beautiful and miraculous efficiency.

A perfect pH

These compounds also regulate the acid-alkaline balance, otherwise known as the blood's pH. The pH of the body is one of the key features in maintaining great health. Maintaining a slightly alkaline pH is key to preventing disease. Having a pH of 7.4 is optimal and between 6.8 to 7.8 is good.

We are living in such stressful times, and trying to find balance in our lives is as difficult as trying to find balance in our bodies. There is much new evidence that our pH levels might have a direct impact on depression and mental health. Studies performed by John Wemmie, MD, PhD, a neuroscientist at the University of Iowa, have uncovered interesting information about how acidity in the brain (pH) may impact brain function. You can speak with your doctor or nutritionist about whether to take probiotics or even small amounts of apple cider vinegar, both of which are thought to help maintain a balanced pH.

Misinformation

Many types of chronic illnesses are the consequence of mis-information passing from malfunctioning cells to healthy cells, which in turn causes cells, organs, and systems to malfunction. Like a virus within your computer, aberrant commands can alter the function of your cells, as well as your body's most elemental form of intelligence—your genes—and thus lead to illness and death.

Cell neighborhoods

The process by which cells communicate with each other is called *signal transduction,* and our understanding of this cellular communication is revolutionizing science.

In order to facilitate communication, groups of cells are arranged in neighborhoods, which are closely monitored and coordinated so that individual cells do not act arbitrarily, or without regard to the overall good of the system. Within those neighborhoods, signals are passed back and forth between cells, instructing some cells to multiply, others to remain inactive, and still others to actually commit suicide.

Once a cell receives a signal from one of its neighbors, new signals are triggered inside the cell. Now a new set of messenger proteins race along pathways within the cell, pathways that are more complex than any subway system ever conceived of by the human imagination. Eventually, the right messenger protein makes its way to specific targets within the cell, but not before the cell has made a set of highly complex decisions about what signals to send, and what genes to stimulate in order to produce just the right action.

If all of this sounds just a bit mind boggling, well, you are glimpsing the dilemma scientists themselves are struggling with every day. Researchers say that it may take many decades before they figure out the vast cellular "wiring diagram" that exists in all of us.

Cells Think!

In order to better understand the process, and how insulin can affect it, we ventured to the laboratory of one of the world's leading specialists in cellular communication, or signal transduction.

The Princeton University campus is dominated by gray, collegiate Gothic architecture, with spires, castle turrets, and gargoyles. These neo-Oxford influences are balanced by many dozens of modern buildings, all of which are low and accessible. The other dominant features of the campus are its trees—they're everywhere—and the many grassy squares and cozy niches, which seem to beckon couples and cohorts to their benches for intimate conversation. To walk across the campus is to be enveloped in an atmosphere that seems infused with the presence of the great thinkers and artists who graced these lawns and buildings—Einstein, Feynman, Toni Morrison, Anthony Burgess, just to name a few.

In one of the campus's more modern structures, the Lewis Thomas Laboratory, you will find one of the world's leading scientists of our day, Jim Broach, PhD, a pioneer in the field of signal transduction, or the study of how cells pass information within and between themselves.

Broach is gray haired and fit. He has the square jaw of a former athlete and small, round eyes that blink frequently when he's trying to formulate his carefully constructed answers. Currently he is a professor and chair of the Department of Biochemistry and Molecular Biology at Penn State College of Medicine, and the director of Penn State Institute for Personalized Medicine. Formerly he was a professor of molecular biology and associate director of the Lewis-Sigler Institute for Integrative Genomics at Princeton, a title that sums up the range of his expertise on the subjects of cell function and gene theory. When Dr. Broach described, in part, the latest scientific understanding of how cells function and maintain health, he began with a startling revelation.

"Cells think," he said matter-of-factly. "They have intelligence. The cell has to take information from multiple inputs and bring them together and balance them out and then decide on a behavior that is informed by all of those different inputs. That processing of information from multiple inputs and then giving an appropriate and coherent response is what I think of as cells thinking."

Though Broach's work occurs primarily in single-cell yeast, much of what he is discovering is also being found in mammalian cells, including our own. "I was surprised to find that one of my colleagues—a colleague with whom I had not discussed this—uses exactly the same term—that cells think. We have found this in yeast cells, and he's found it in mammalian cells. But it's exactly the same idea."

Cells Make Decisions

Right now, for example, your cells are being bombarded by an enormous volume of information that is flowing in your bloodstream. They are evaluating, for example, the availability of oxygen, protein, and nutrition, the presence of disease-causing agents, the blood's temperature, the availability of fuel, and the level of insulin that's present in the blood. Elsewhere in the body, nerve cells are sensing your clothing, your weight on the chair, the temperature in the room you are sitting in, and the availability of oxygen in that room. Cells in your eyes are converting the light images that emerge from this page into nerve impulses that are sent on to your brain, enabling you to read. In each instance, your cells are making decisions about how to respond to the stimuli with which they are being bombarded.

"The decisions a cell makes determine whether you maintain health or whether your body is thrown off homeostasis, such as when you suffer from a disease such as diabetes," said Dr. Broach.

Passing on the message

Understanding that cells think is a recent insight for scientists. Not only do cells weigh information and give an intelligent response, but they also communicate that response within themselves—that is, to targets within the cell, such as specific genes—and then to other cells within the larger organism.

But the challenge to communicate effectively within organs—composed of millions of cells—and to the body at large, composed of trillions of them, is beyond comprehension. Understanding how this remarkable feat is accomplished is the task that Dr. Broach, and other scientists like him, have set for themselves.

One cell becomes three trillion

Like all multicellular animals, each of us developed from a single cell that doubled, and then kept doubling. At five days after conception, we were little more than a tiny embryonic dot, no bigger than the period at the end of this sentence. From that repeated doubling of cells came a fully formed human being. Such a feat was made possible, in part, by the ability of our cells to specialize, or differentiate, into some 200 different varieties. Hundreds of millions of cells took on specialized abilities to form the brain, others the heart, and still others the digestive tract, reproductive organs, arms and hands, legs and feet. Like good basketball players, our cells took up their positions and matured, each contributing to the body parts, organs, etc. that make up a human being.

Group work

Of course, that was just the beginning. The estimated three trillion cells that make up your body must cooperate with each other if the human body is to form, and health is to be maintained. In order for this to happen, cells must communicate. Groups of cells begin to work in close contact with each other, like neighborhoods, with each community exerting a kind of social control over its members. No cell, for example, is allowed to multiply without express instructions from its neighbors. Those same neighbors also tell the cell when to stop multiplying and enter a more quiet or restful phase. The same is true for many other cellular functions.

Lone cell

Every time a cell starts to act independently the entire organism is in jeopardy.

Cancer is but one example. Essentially, cancer is a disease characterized by cells that mutate—or undergo genetic changes—causing them to reproduce continually. Neighboring cells command malignant cells to shut down and even to self-destruct, but unfortunately, cancer cells become disassociated from the signals from others cells. Instead of shutting down, the cancer cells continue to replicate without regard to the health of the overall organism. The result is the overpopulation of certain types of cells that use up vital resources, yet do not perform vital tasks. They are autonomous tumors, gobbling up the blood and oxygen of the body, while ignoring signals from neighboring cells to cease growing. Cancer is a disease that arises when cell communication breaks down.

Messengers

Cells communicate with each other, says Dr. Broach, by passing messages back and forth in the form of protein molecules, also known as *cytokines*. Each cytokine gives a specific set of orders to neighboring cells, or sometimes to those at a distance. Cells can receive messages because they are equipped with a specialized receptor—think of it as a baseball player's glove—that is itself composed of protein.

Signals

Though proteins are the primary source of communication between cells, other specialized cells can create different types of signals. Endocrine cells, for example, create and send hormones such as insulin, testosterone, and estrogen, which travel through the bloodstream and can target distant cells. Nerve cells, known as neurons, create chemicals known as *neurotransmitters* that give rise to moods and mental states, such as optimism or depression, relaxation or alertness. Neurons also rely on electrical signals that fire within and between the nerve cells.

Once a cell receives a hormone, cytokine, or neurotransmitter, it initiates another series of internal messengers within itself. These messengers relay information to different stops on pathways toward an ultimate goal—oftentimes a specific gene, or set of genes, within the cell's headquarters, or nucleus.

Protein kinases and baseball

Within cells, the messenger proteins that travel along the cell's inner pathways are enzymes known as *kinases*. So far, scientists have identified as many as 500 kinases. These proteins act as catalysts, either turning on a cell function or turning it off. Not only are there hundreds of kinases, but they often also undergo changes that further refine or alter their commands. One of the primary ways kinases are altered is through a process called *phosphorylation*, which chemically and electrically alters the kinase's signal so that it can activate or inhibit a specific cellular activity.

The process is not unlike a basic ground ball to third base. Once the original signaling molecule is caught, it is then fired to, say, second base, which passes it on to first, and then home. In the cell, these pathways are infinitely complex, with many different stops along the way. However, if the pH is off balance and the insulin irregular, then the communication between cells is "Who is on first?" "What's on second?" and "I don't know on third" (with thanks to Abbott and Costello).

Lightning-speed information

The human body is ablaze with crisscrossing lines of information, flowing within cells and between them, at breathtaking speeds. The transfer of information from the tip of your toe to your brain can occur at speeds of 100 meters per second. This speed is one of the reasons we can recognize an oncoming car barreling down the street, assess the danger, and quickly move out of its way—all in a matter of milliseconds. Now imagine those same speeds occurring within a microscopic-sized cell, and you begin to get an idea of the level of difficulty involved in mapping the inner pathways of cells.

Wiring

Not only do scientists have to contend with the speed with which information flows, but also the body's vastly complex inner circuitry, referred to as the "wiring diagram." At one point in our discussion with Dr. Broach, he took out a scientific journal that contained a drawing of only some of the pathways that are known to exist within a single cell. Those pathways were so complex that they resembled the London subway system—only *doubled*.

To make matters even more challenging—and delicate—a cell receives not just one signal at a time, but many all at once. If we use our baseball analogy again, we might say that it isn't just one ground ball to third base, but literally dozens of ground balls being fired to dozens of bases, all at the same time—and all the players getting it right!

Cell Intelligence

"For many years," said Jim Broach, "we as biologists have been studying how any one signal impinges on and changes the behavior of a cell. And we have learned that different signals change the cell in different ways. Some signals tell the cell to grow; some tell it to stop growing. What we are learning now is that the cell doesn't get a single signal, but multiple signals at the same time, and it has to decide what is the appropriate response at that moment."

Which brings us to an even deeper mystery that, as yet, cannot be fully explained. Some form of intelligence, buried deeply within cells, is organizing each cell's response to the incoming information. That intelligence is the true source of your physical, emotional, and intellectual health.

Transcription factors

Though we don't fully understand this organizing intelligence, scientists do know at least one place from which it functions—a tiny array of proteins known as *transcription factors*. These transcription factors regulate the functioning of genes, in effect turning specific genes on and off.

Transcription factors are located around our DNA and are constantly issuing commands to our genes. We have between 20,000 and 30,000 genes, which contain our biological inheritance. Transcription factors are signaling those genes to produce specific proteins, such as muscle proteins, or immune proteins that destroy disease and maintain your health.

Unlike a computer, which does little more than accept incoming data, transcription factors receive the information and then make precise decisions in order to produce the best and most appropriate response to the event. Transcription factors, for example, will determine which signals to send within the cell, which pathways those signals will travel upon, and which genes will be expressed, or shut down. It does this by sending kinases along specific pathways to targeted genes.

Transcription factors also order the cell to send out signals to other cells to form a coordinated response in the body.

Genes: instruments in the grand symphony

The role of transcription factors and their effects on our genes disabuses us of one of the more popular cultural beliefs, which is that genes are the ultimate arbiters of our fate. In reality, genes are more like instruments in a grand symphony, each one waiting for the moment when the maestro will point the baton and call forth its music. Genes determine a great deal of our underlying nature, but transcription factors—the cellular maestros—are triggering your genes or keeping them quiet. The delicate virtuosity with which your cells are able to express each relevant gene—and do it at just the right moment—determines your health, and indeed your fate.

"Think of transcription factors as a kind of aristocracy within the cell," Dr. Broach says. "Not only are they taking in and balancing lots of information, and making a decision about that information, but they are also regulating a large number of genes"—sometimes as many as 50 genes or more. Once the transcription factor makes its decision, it sends a kinase to trigger a particular gene or group of genes.

For example, transcription factors trigger just such a sequence when you experience pain. Following a bodily injury, there is an increase in the activity of certain transcription factors located in the spinal cord and sensory neurons. These transcription factors stimulate the production of specific molecules that increase inflammatory proteins and generate pain signaling to the brain. Your body knows that it has been injured because transcription factors are passing along that information to your brain.

Hormones send signals

Many hormones play a critical role in the vast majority of cell signaling. Insulin is an extremely important one. When balanced, insulin facilitates the smooth flow of information and overall health. But when insulin becomes chronically elevated, or when insulin resistance sets in, breakdowns occur—throughout the body and its systems.

(For example insulin, to a great extent, determines your body weight and, more specifically, how much fatty tissue your body carries around. The more insulin is in your blood, the fatter you become. The fatter you are, the larger your fat cells become. The bigger your fat cells the more likely it is that something will go wrong.

Fat cells are highly active tissues, producing a variety of chemicals, most of which are detrimental to your health. Among the more damaging of those chemicals are cytokines that promote inflammation throughout the body, thus increasing your chances of getting heart disease, high blood pressure, diabetes, cancer, arthritis, asthma, and other inflammatory illnesses. These poisonous cytokines also stimulate increased cell division and cancer.)

In an insulin-resistant environment, cells grow new and different types of receptors that make them highly sensitive to insulin in the bloodstream. In a high-insulin environment, those receptors are constantly being stimulated, signaling cells to divide, multiply, and proliferate, often without regard for their neighbors, or for the good of the body as a whole, thus dramatically increasing the likelihood of developing some form of cancer.

Certain types of cancers, such as colon cancer, display excessive amounts of receptors for insulin, a fact that has causes scientists to theorize that cancer cells depend upon an increase in insulin signaling to promote tumor growth. Many researchers now believe that insulin may feed cancer cells.

In addition to producing poisonous cytokines, fatty tissues also pump out great volumes of sex hormones, such as estrogen, which can also serve as cancer promoters. Estrogen is not cancerous in and of itself, but metabolites of estrogen—the byproducts of estrogen utilization by the body—can stimulate the growth of cancer.

Command to Destruct!

As if all of this were not enough, insulin resistance can also change the way kinases behave, which in turn can damage the cell's DNA, thus preventing cells from responding to neighboring cells' commands. One of the great decisions that cellular neighborhoods have to make is to order a cell, or groups of cells, to commit what biologists refer to as *apoptosis*, or "programmed cell death." Every cell is equipped with a self-destruct sequence, which is an essential program that enables the body to rid itself of potentially harmful cells. In a system that is continually striving for homeostasis, there is no room for unneeded cells.

Eliminating cells

The body must eliminate cells that do not mature or differentiate, or do not perform any needed task, but instead take up space and consume needed resources. These vagrant cells also pose a threat to the system, because they can become cancerous. Indeed, cancer is an ever-growing group of cells that do not differentiate, but instead gobble up resources and turn healthy organs into nonfunctioning masses of tissue.

Insulin resistance often leads to the increased production of growth hormone, which in turn corrodes the gene inside of cells that is responsible for triggering apoptosis. Thus, when the neighborhood cells recognize that one of their cohort is growing out of control, they tell the renegade cell, or cells, to initiate programmed cell death. But thanks to the effects of growth hormone, the mutant cells have broken free of the neighborhood's constraints and can act independently, without regard for the overall organism.

Apoptosis: the right amount of cell death

Let's get our brain cells going. Do you remember that one word from high school biology—"apoptosis"? Well here is what it's all about. The body relies on apoptosis to maintain overall organ function and integrity. Indeed, during fetal development, when organs are rapidly being formed, the body uses apoptosis to "sculpt" organs, cleaving away unneeded tissue. This is especially important in the brain, with its highly complex regions and geography—the cerebrum, cerebellum, limbic system, and hypothalamus, for example. When the fetus is growing inside the mother's womb, cells are multiplying within the blink of an eye. Apoptosis helps to keep each of the brain's regions in correct proportion to each other. It also helps to maintain the brain's structural integrity throughout life, as it does for every other organ in the body.

Unfortunately, high insulin levels may interfere with

this process. New research is now showing that chronically high insulin during fetal development interferes with apoptosis and thus allows parts of the brain to grow disproportionately large.

As you can easily see, getting just the right amount of apoptosis—without destroying essential organs—is a delicate feat, one that depends on precise communication between and within cells.

Insulin, cell death, and the brain

Just as high insulin and insulin resistance can block apoptosis from occurring in some cells, it can also trigger unwanted cell death in others. Much to our horror, insulin resistance in the brain can stimulate unwanted apoptosis in neurons, causing whole swaths of brain cells to destroy themselves and thus bring on memory loss, dementia, and Alzheimer's disease. New research is now showing that Alzheimer's may be a form of "diabetes of the brain."

When brain levels of insulin remain high, neurons begin sending out messengers that trigger apoptosis in brain cells. Cells initiate programmed cell death. Many brain functions degrade and vast swaths of memory are lost, forming the basis for Alzheimer's disease.

Chronically high insulin can interfere with the balance of neurotransmitters in the brain, thus forming the basis for an array of other mental and emotional imbalances, especially in children.

Possible connection to autism

Some researchers now believe that this failure of apoptosis may play a role in the onset of autism.

Several recent studies have shown abnormally high levels of insulin-related growth factors in the spinal fluid of children with autism. Researchers point out that a precise balance of these growth factors is essential for normal brain development. However, when insulin-related growth factors become abnormally high, this delicate balance is disturbed, causing certain parts of the brain to become overly developed—the very abnormalities we see in children with autism. Please be aware that this is just one possible factor amongst thousands of possible scientific explanations for autism.

Robust health and dynamic body balance (also known as *homeostasis*) depends on the efficient communication of the trillions of your body's cells. The disruption or miscommunication of a cell (or a neighborhood of cells) is the very beginning of any illness or disease.

Insulin signaling is involved in the multiple epidemics we face today, including overweight, obesity, heart disease, certain cancers, attention deficit disorders in children, and an explosion of neurological diseases, including Alzheimer's. At face value, all of these illnesses look distinctly different from one another. But as scientists investigate the illnesses' deeper origins, they are discovering that illnesses spring from the same underlying source of systems biology, including insulin resistance, inflammation, pH imbalance and mitochondrial dysfunction, destroying the lives of both young and old.

CHAPTER 4

Insulin Resistance Metabolic Syndrome, and Diabetes

Bill's story

Bill Diamond, married and the father of three, was 39 years old and 50 pounds overweight. His cholesterol level was dangerously high at 250 mg/dl, and his triglycerides (or blood fats) were even worse, at 270 mg/dl. He had heart disease, high blood pressure, respiratory distress, and gout, a form of arthritis common among those who eat a high-fat, high-protein diet. He also suffered occasional chest pains. Finally, his fasting blood glucose level was 125 mg/dl, which meant that he was borderline diabetic. His doctor had already told him that he was "insulin resistant," meaning that his cells were so stuffed with blood sugar that they were trying to block any more fuel from entering.

(When cells try to refuse to accept blood sugar, or glucose, it means that there will be an overabundance of sugar in the blood, a dangerous condition that can lead to brain swelling, diabetic coma, and death.)

Bill's body was reacting to his insulin resistance by producing even more insulin, which was forcing the glucose into his cells. But that only made the cells more inflamed.

"Bill," his doctor said. "Diabetes has been shown to shorten a person's life by 15 years on average. I'm giving you all the drugs we have and they're not reversing the condition. If you keep going like this, you're never going to see 65."

There are almost 30 million diabetics in the United States. The vast majority—25 million—have what is called type 2 diabetes, which arises when the body no longer uses insulin properly. The vast majority of these people are insulin resistant. In China the most recent estimate is that at least 12%, or 115 million people, are living with diabetes, and possibly three to four times that number with prediabetes and metabolic syndrome. Typical treatment for insulin resistance and type 2 diabetes includes weight loss, changes in diet, and—if these measures fail, which they often do—medication.

Type 1 diabetes occurs when the pancreas can no longer produce insulin. Because insulin is essential for life, these people must take insulin injections in order to survive.

So much damage

All diabetics, no matter which form of diabetes they may

suffer from, are far more likely than healthy adults to experience an array of terrible side effects, including heart disease, high blood pressure, erectile dysfunction, retinal eye damage, potential blindness, kidney disease, even gangrene and loss of limbs. Diabetes is the number one cause of loss of limbs and blindness in the US.

Prediabetes

There are possibly 86 million Americans who are prediabetic, meaning that they have high insulin levels and are overweight, and therefore are at high risk of contracting the illness. Prediabetics also have an increased risk of suffering from the same related disorders that diabetics do.

Insulin resistance is the foundation of the vast majority of diabetes cases in the world. And what most Americans do not realize is that they are eating their way toward this terrible scourge with every meal.

From your plate into your cells

When you eat a meal, the nutrients in that meal are absorbed by your small intestine and then into your bloodstream. Once in your blood, the carbohydrates from your meal are converted into sugar molecules, now called *glucose*, which is your body's preferred fuel. The fat in your meal becomes fatty acids, or triglycerides, in your blood. These triglycerides are stored in your tissues as fat, which is a future source of energy in the event that calorie consumption falls.

Your brain recognizes the arrival of glucose in your system and responds by telling your pancreas to produce insulin. Once secreted, insulin flows to your cells, where it binds with, and stimulates, a specialized insulin-receptor on the cell membrane. That in turn triggers a kinase (enzyme) cascade inside the cell membrane that allows glucose to enter the cells. Additional kinases are then triggered, which carry the glucose to the cell's mitochondria, the furnace inside your cells that transforms glucose into adenosine triphosphate, or ATP, the substance your cells can use as energy.

Gas tank is full

Like the gas tank and engine in your car, your cells have a limit to how much fuel they can absorb. If you pump too much gas into your car's tank, the gas will overflow onto the ground. While your car is not going to be affected by the attempt to put in more gas than it can handle, that's not the case with your body. The worst consequence of too much glucose in your bloodstream is diabetic coma and death. Consequently, your brain monitors your blood sugar levels very carefully, and will do all it can to bring glucose levels into the normal ranges as quickly as it can.

Burn up or weigh down

When we eat a meal that's rich in calories—calories from fat or from carbohydrates—glucose levels rise rapidly in the blood. The brain recognizes this as an emergency situation and immediately sets two strategies in motion in order to save your life. First, it attempts to burn as much of the blood sugar as it can. The only place it can do that is inside your cells. Therefore, the brain signals the pancreas to produce more insulin, which forces the excess glucose into the cells, where it will be burned as fuel.

The second strategy is to store as much of the glucose as it can in your muscles, liver, and fatty tissues, known as adipose tissue.

In order to be stored in your liver and muscles, glucose must be converted to a substance called *glycogen*, which is utilized as fuel whenever glucose levels fall. The remaining glucose will be converted to fatty acids, known as triglycerides, and stored as fat.

Too many carbohydrates become fat on your body because they are converted to triglycerides, a form of fat, and then stored on your stomach, buttocks, legs, and other parts of your body as fatty tissue. Elevated blood triglycerides stimulate your liver to produce more cholesterol, which increases the risk of heart attack and stroke.

Shut down

While these changes are going on in your liver, muscles, and fat tissue, your cells are being force-fed the excess glucose that's in your blood, a situation they cannot endure for long. When this situation persists, your cells close their insulin receptors in order to shut off the flow of fuel. When cells stop accepting glucose, they suffer from a condition doctors refer to as "insulin resistance."

Effects of Insulin Resistance

Insulin resistance and metabolic syndrome can cause bio-chemical changes that may form the basis for an array of serious illnesses in general, and diabetes in particular.

- *Blood cholesterol* levels increase eventually, causing tissues throughout the body to become inflamed and swollen with cholesterol plaque, including the arteries that lead to the heart and brain. Such conditions, of course, form the basis for a heart attack or stroke.
- *High levels of inflammation*, which, among other things, cause the tiny nephrons in the kidneys to become blocked with plaque, reducing their ability to filter and cleanse the blood, a function essential to life.
- *Weight may increase*, leading to the production of hormones that promote even greater weight gain.

Complications of Diabetes

- *Circulation of blood is reduced* throughout the system. Fingers and toes may become numb and prone to infection, nerve damage, and even gan-grene. Eventually, this can lead to amputation.
- Many diabetics eventually develop *kidney dysfunction* or even kidney failure, resulting in the need for dialysis to remain alive.
- When blood flow to the reproductive organs is

impeded, *erectile dysfunction* is common. This is common in diabetics.

- *Retinal damage* in the eye is common in long-standing diabetics due to the narrowing of the tiny blood vessels of the retina.
- There is some evidence suggesting that there may be a link to *certain cancers* such as breast, colon, and prostate.

Metabolic Syndrome

Elevated triglycerides, cholesterol, hormones, and weight combine to create what is called "metabolic syndrome," a prediabetic condition that can lead to high blood pressure, heart disease, stroke, diabetes, disorders of the joints, circulatory problems, erectile dysfunction impotence, and possibly even certain types of cancers.

Disrupts cell signals

Insulin resistance and metabolic syndrome can affect every aspect of our biology, for the simple reason that it disrupts the signaling that occurs within cells. Once the signaling is broken down, cells themselves function in aberrant and destructive ways, which of course leads to illness. Insulin resistance in the brain can cause the signaling within neurons to become disrupted.

Unfortunately, insulin resistance forces the body to produce more and more insulin in order to get the cells to accept the glucose in your blood.

In his book, *How Fat Works* (Harvard University Press, 2009), Philip A. Wood, D.V.M., PhD, director of the integrative metabolism program at Lake Nona, and former director of the division of genomics at the University of Alabama, describes insulin resistance this way: "The difference between a healthy person and one who is insulin resistant is that a healthy person immediately experiences a drop in blood glucose levels after his or her body produces insulin. The person who is insulin resistant, however, experiences no significant drop in blood sugar levels, even after his or her body produces significant amounts of insulin." In essence, the blood is still flooded with glucose after a meal—a dangerous condition. The body can only react to this situation by producing even more insulin, which will force the cells to accept the glucose. The increase in insulin will also cause the body to convert the glucose into fat and store it as rapidly as possible.

Dr. Wood goes on to explain that "insulin resistance is defined as the condition whereby the body's cells require more and more insulin to get the same effect of glucose uptake."

Insulin resistance is the basis for the onset of diabetes, though most people are insulin resistant for a decade or more before they actually contract diabetes. If you develop a metabolic syndrome—which means high glucose, high triglycerides, and high insulin—for long enough, you may well contract type 2 diabetes.

Type 2 diabetics produce higher than normal quantities of insulin, but also require oral medication to stabilize their blood sugar. Nevertheless, the pancreas will have to produce more and more insulin in order to keep pace with the high levels of glucose in the bloodstream. Eventually, the pancreas will give out and lose its ability to produce insulin entirely. At that point, insulin injections will be needed and the person will develop insulin-dependent diabetes.

Three central factors

Essentially, there are three factors that lead to insulin resistance—the kinds of foods we eat, our exercise habits (or the lack of them), and our genetic make-up. Researchers are quick to point out, however, that even if you are genetically susceptible to insulin resistance and diabetes, you can avoid both disorders by following a healthy lifestyle.

As an example, scientists point to the Pima tribe of Arizona, who have the highest rates of Type 2 diabetes and obesity on earth. Yet their genetically similar cousins, the Pimas of Northern Mexico, experience extremely low rates of diabetes and obesity, though they too possess the same genetic vulnerability to both disorders. In fact, the two tribes actually originated from the same peoples, who migrated from Asia and settled in North American some 30,000 years ago. One part of the tribe made their home in Arizona, while the other went to northern Mexico. Researchers who have studied the two tribes closely have shown that their different disease patterns arise from their very different diets and exercise patterns. The Pimas of Arizona eat a diet that is rich in fat and calories, and lead largely sedentary lives. The Pimas of Mexico eat a diet made up largely of whole grains, vegetables, beans, and small quantities of animal protein. They work hard physically and enjoy various kinds of traditional sports.

These two Pima communities reveal what is happening throughout the United States and around the world—people are eating too many calories and engaging in too little exercise. That's a lethal combination.

We were never meant to eat this much!

The Harvard Medical School in Boston is just a few miles from the more well-known, picturesque campus in Cambridge, which is just across the Charles River. They might as well be two different worlds. The ivy-strewn red brick buildings that are the trademark of the Cambridge campus are nowhere to be seen at the medical school. Here the buildings are gray and tan fortresses, intimidating and blatantly heartless. They are short on art and long on message—an imposing one at that. *We do serious work here,* these buildings seem to say, *and when we look at you, we look with a cold eye.*

On the eighth floor of the Beth Israel Deaconess Medical Center at Harvard Medical School you will find George Blackburn, MD, PhD, one of the world's leading experts on insulin resistance, cardiovascular disease, and diabetes.

"We were never meant to eat this many calories," he said. "It's too much for the body. If you look back at the wisdom of our ancestors, you will find that they knew that overeating was bad for your health. They knew to eat smaller meals and to chew the food thoroughly. That was just common sense. Today, it seems we've forgotten a lot of that ancient wisdom."

One of the consequences of our amnesia is insulin resistance, said Blackburn, and all the problems that go with it.

The fat story

"It all begins with fatty acids," he said. "Circulating fatty acids get into the machinery of the cell and block the kinases within the cell. Basically, overeating saturated fat and calories causes the cell to become disrupted and brings on insulin resistance."

Blackburn explained that the fat in our diets are converted in the body to triglycerides, which are composed of three fatty acids riding on the back of an alcohol molecule called a glycerol. Triglycerides come from two sources—the fat in our foods, and the excess calories we consume.

There are drugs to lower triglycerides, Dr. Blackburn pointed out, but they are not going to have the same effect as simply limiting the amount of fat we eat, especially saturated fat and an artificially produced fat called trans fats.

There are four forms of dietary fat—saturated, trans fats, polyunsaturated, and monounsaturated fats. By far, the most poisonous are saturated and trans fats, both of which are solid at room temperature, thanks to the fact that both are filled to capacity with hydrogen atoms. Both saturated and trans fats raise blood cholesterol levels, especially the bad cholesterol known as low-density lipoproteins (LDL). Saturated fat is found primarily in animal foods, such as red meat, dairy products, eggs, and chicken. Trans fats are made by food manufacturers who harden vegetable oils—liquid at room temperature—by infusing them with hydrogen atoms, thus turning them into saturated fats.

Saturated fats and trans fats are more likely to promote insulin resistance and other illnesses, including heart disease. One of the ways they do this is by causing the liver to become inflamed and disrupting signaling within liver cells. The liver plays a central role in insulin resistance, especially when it has been overfed with lots of fatty acids.

Polyunsaturated fats, which come from vegetable and fish oils, are liquid at room temperature. They lower total blood cholesterol and LDL and offer some protection against heart disease. Monounsaturated fats, which come primarily from olive oil and are also liquid at room temperature, have no effect on LDL, but may raise HDL, the good cholesterol, and thus may also offer some protection against heart disease. Monounsaturated fats also reduce the size of fat cells and promote weight loss.

Consumption of poly- and monounsaturated fats are associated with lower rates of all illnesses, including diabetes. People who follow a Mediterranean diet, for example, have far lower rates of metabolic syndrome, diabetes, heart disease, and many forms of cancer. They tend to eat relatively more olive oil, and significantly less animal products and saturated fats. They also eat dramatically lower levels of trans fats, which are found primarily in processed foods. There is good evidence to show that poly- and monounsaturated fats may also reduce inflammation, thus protecting against a number of serious illnesses.

As recently as November 2016, in a *Nature Journal*

article, researchers at the Washington University School of Medicine in St. Louis have identified a possible trigger of chronic inflammation. Dr. Clay Semenkovich and Dr. Michael Karl discovered that a high fat diet seems to be the trigger for inflammation.

The interesting aspect of this study is that the inflammation seems to be caused by the macrophages synthesizing fat in the cells. When this process is blocked by inhibiting the enzyme for fatty acid synthesis in these immune cells, no inflammation occurs. This data confirms that sugar alone is not the culprit in insulin resistance and type 2 diabetes; it is in fact a high fat diet. These findings will be important for other conditions such as arthritis and cancer.

What is a calorie?

Fat is the most calorically dense substance in the food supply. A gram of fat provides nine calories, while a gram of protein and carbohydrate contain only four. A calorie is a unit of potential energy found in food. The more calories we consume, the more potential energy our bodies possess. However, the calories that are not burned as fuel are turned into fatty acids in our blood, and thus can disrupt cell signaling and lead to insulin resistance.

Concentrated calories

By far, the biggest source of calories in our diets is processed food, and the more processed, the greater the concentration of the calories in the food. Processed foods include rolls, pastries, bread, cookies, muffins, cakes, candy, soda, and processed cheeses and meats, such as bologna, sausage, and pepperoni. These foods are extremely dense in calories. In essence, food manufacturers take a great quantity of natural foods, such as corn or wheat or potatoes, grind them up, dry them out, cook them down, and turn them into a smaller volume of food. Processing causes carbohydrates to become concentrated, which means that processed foods are going to cause weight gain.

In his book, *The Pritikin Principle: The Calorie Density Solution* (Time-Life Books, 2000), Robert Pritikin shows what happens in the process. A pound of corn, for example, provides 390 calories. But a pound of cornflakes provides 1,770 calories. The same thing happens to potatoes, which provides about 490 calories per pound. A pound of potato chips, however, gives us 2400 calories. Now the truth is, you probably couldn't eat a pound of potatoes, at least not in a single sitting, because potatoes are loaded with fiber and water, which provide bulk, and thus fill you up, but contain no calories. Yet plenty of people—especially teenagers—eat a pound of potato chips without blinking an eye. (A common container for potato and corn chips is a one-pound bag.)

Nutrient dense

Natural, unprocessed grains—such as brown rice, millet, barley, quinoa, and whole wheat berries—are rich in complex carbohydrates, which are slowly absorbed and do not create spikes in insulin levels. The same is true for other plant sources of carbohydrates, such as squash, turnips, broccoli, and other pulpy vegetables. Not only are the carbs in these foods slowly absorbed, but these foods are also essentially low in calories. A pound of brown rice—far more than you could eat in a single meal, or even in a single day—has less than 500 calories. A pound of broccoli, again more than you could eat in a single sitting, has about 85 calories.

But process the carbohydrates in, say, whole wheat, and you can produce a pound or more of bread, which contains about 1200 calories. When you go to a supermarket today and look down the aisles, most of the foods you see are processed, which means most of them will cause weight gain. You can avoid processed foods by switching to a diet that contains more vegetables, fruit, and cooked, whole, and unprocessed grains. Another way to lower the calorie content of your diet is to avoid sugar-rich soft drinks.

Lethal soft drinks!

Coca Cola, Mountain Dew, Dr. Pepper, Sprite and 7-Up: these drinks are little more than "liquid candy," says Michael Jacobson, PhD, director of the Center for Science in the Public Interest (CSPI). The average 12-ounce can of soda contains 10 teaspoons of pure sugar (the equivalent of 40 grams), and 160 calories. (The large Coke sold by McDonalds contains 310 calories.) Needless to say, there is no nutritional value in these drinks, which means that the calories are empty. Most fruit juice is just as bad, mostly packed with masses of added sugar. Even 100% pure juices contain such refined and quickly absorbable sugar content that it causes the same insulin response as a can of coke.

On average, Americans consume at least two soft drinks per day, or 48 gallons of soda pop a year, CSPI reports. According to the *American Journal of Clinical Nutrition*, carbonated soft drinks are the single biggest source of refined sugar in the American diet.

"Teens just about hit their recommended sugar limits from soft drinks alone," says Dr. Jacobson. "With candy, cookies, cake, ice cream, and other sugary foods, most exceed those recommendations by a large margin." It's common for children and teenagers to wash down snacks with soft drinks.

This is the problem facing American youths today: they're consuming sugar, soda, and processed foods throughout every day of their lives. Not only do many schools have vending machines in their hallways that dispense nothing but processed, sugar-rich foods, but at the same time, the school cafeterias serve an abundance of these same fat- and calorie-rich foods at every noonday meal. The average child's social life is built on calorie-rich sweets.

Consider the ever-escalating trend in children's birthday parties—the "goodie bag syndrome." Our kids spend the entire afternoon eating cake, cookies, pizza, soda, ice tea, and candy, and then are sent home with a bag full of treats—the "goodie bag"—for later in the evening. They're mainlining sugar and calories. Parents feel they must ply the kids with sugar if the party is to be successful. In an average grammar school class, there are between 20 and 30 parties throughout the school year. Is it any wonder that so many children are overweight and addicted to sugar and processed foods? If this trend continues, it will not take a crystal ball to figure out that our children's future, and the future of our country, is an adulthood dominated by illness.

The US is not alone. This is a global epidemic. In their book entitled *Fat China: How Expanding Waistlines are Changing a Nation*, Paul French and Matthew Crabbe explain how, in a decade, there has been a sharp rise in soft drink consumption amongst the Chinese population. The younger generation in particular has enthusiastically embraced the fast food marketing-led consumer culture. This has created a dire situation, adding to the already numerous causes of rising childhood obesity among urban Chinese and spreading to more and more cities and country regions.

What is a glycemic index (GI)?

Processed foods have a very different effect on glucose and insulin levels than unprocessed foods do. In an unprocessed, natural food, such as squash or brown rice, the carbohydrates are bound up in long chains that are woven into the food's fibers. Those carbohydrates must be worked on by the intestines so that they can be freed from the fiber and long molecular chains. Little by little these carbohydrates are broken free and released into your bloodstream, giving you a long-lasting supply of glucose, but keeping insulin levels relatively low.

This is what is meant by a low GI (glycemic index). The glucose gets absorbed very slowly and has a gentle effect on insulin and the pancreas.

Something very different happens when you eat a processed food. Processing extracts the carbohydrates from their fibrous chains, turning those complex carbs into simple sugars. Once that's done, the sugars are concentrated in much smaller volumes of food, as are typically found in candy, cakes, or soft drinks—or high GI foodstuffs. Some of these simple sugars flow into your bloodstream while they are still in your mouth, requiring very little energy for your body to process them. Those that do make it to your small intestine require no breakdown of fiber and no real digestion. These too are rapidly absorbed into your bloodstream. Not only are these sugars quickly absorbed, but they also arrive in enormous quantities. It's as if your blood is suddenly flooded with simple sugars, which sends your blood sugar and insulin levels skyrocketing. That, of course, propels the body into an emergency situation in which it must lower its glucose levels as quickly as possible.

Force-feeding your cells!

As glucose floods the blood, the body immediately responds with a spike in insulin levels and cells are force-fed glucose. Meanwhile, the body tries to store quantities of blood sugar, first in the muscles, and then in the liver. The muscles, which are huge repositories for stored fuel, convert as much glucose into glycogen—the stored form of fuel—as they can. The problem is that if you are insulin resistant, or diabetic, your muscles are already packed with unused glycogen. In essence, their fuel tanks are full, which means they can no longer accept additional fuel, or glucose, into their cells. Meanwhile, lack of exercise causes inactive muscle tissue to lose its ability to utilize glucose, as well as convert glucose into glycogen, or stored fuel. There's little or no need for stored fuel in muscle tissue that's not burning much fuel to begin with.

In fact, the inability of insulin-resistant muscles to transform glucose into glycogen is severe. The primary defect in insulin action in patients with type 2 diabetes resides in the skeletal muscle. In the study published in *Diabetes Care* in November 2009, DeFronzo and Tripathy demonstrated that muscle glucose uptake is reduced by about 50% in type 2 diabetes.

Exercise: emptying the surplus reserves

In all probability, the reason is simply that the muscles are already chock-full of glycogen, in part because they have not been exercised. Compounding this problem is that insulin-resistant or diabetic individuals often tend to avoid exercise and lead sedentary lives. Muscles need to be exercised in order to burn off, or empty, their glycogen reserves. Without exercise, muscles remain full of reserve fuel. Like their cell counterparts, they cannot take in excess glucose that shows up in the blood. The consequence is that the blood continues to be flooded with glucose, requiring higher levels of insulin to force glucose into cells.

In the face of rising glucose levels, the liver transforms blood sugar into fatty acids to be stored in the adipose tissues as additional fat. This process will add weight to your body. You're not only getting fatter, but your blood is still flooded with both glucose and fatty acids.

Can you reverse insulin resistance?

The excess fat in the adipose tissue is a reservoir for tri-glycerides. "Fatty acids are quickly stored in the tissues," said Dr. Blackburn, "but they are also released rapidly into the bloodstream, as well. The blood is flooded with harm-ful fatty acids."

Many of us think of the fatty tissue around our waist, buttocks, and elsewhere as largely inactive matter, but that is far from the case. The cells in adipose tissue produce hormones and messenger proteins, called cytokines, that regulate numerous cellular functions. When these mes-sengers are produced in balanced quantities, cell function often remains normal. But in overweight people, adipose tissue can overproduce both, which in turn can disrupt cellular function and lead to insulin resistance and other disorders. This is one of the reasons why losing weight is often associated with the elimination of insulin resistance. Weight loss reduces adipose tissue and brings hormones and cytokines more into balance. But you have to lose the weight first before you experience a reduction in these dan-gerous cytokines.

It's worth noting that the current diet and levels of overweight among people are unlike anything we as humans have ever experienced in our two million years of evolution. Processed foods, with their enormous number of calories, are a completely modern phenomenon, and it is only in the last 40 years that they have begun to dominate the diet. Our bodies were not designed for an overabundance—and overconsumption—of food, especially when it is sustained, day in and day out.

We are designed for famine

Far more common in human experience are food shortages and famines, for which the body has adapted protective mechanisms.

One of those protective methods is a process called *gluconeogenesis*, which is the ability of the liver to transform amino acids into fuel, or glucose. When food supplies drop, and glucose levels fall, the liver will first burn its own glycogen reserves. But when they run out, the liver will convert amino acids into glucose, thus keeping the body alive. When the liver is creating new glucose (which is what "gluconeogenesis" means), it is burning fatty acids as fuel. When food is found, and glucose levels rise again, the liver shuts off gluconeogenesis and burns glucose again, thus keeping blood glucose levels normal.

That's how things function in a healthy state. But in an insulin-resistant state, the liver produces more glucose on its own. There's already too much glucose and too many fatty acids in the blood, and now the liver is adding to the burden. This, of course, forces the pancreas to produce even more insulin in order to force glucose into the cells.

The function of insulin receptors

Like finely tuned antennae, the insulin receptors on cells are highly sensitive. Inside the receptor, two delicate protein kinases known as IRS-1 and IRS-2 (IRS for "insulin receptor substrate") await their orders from the insulin. Under healthy conditions, these two molecules, when phosphorylated by insulin, activate a pivotal kinase within the cell known as PI-3 (phosphatidylinositol-3). PI-3, in turn, sets off an entire chain reaction downstream that ensures the smooth flow of glucose from the blood to the appropriate sites within the cell. However, when the blood is too rich in fats, IRS-1, IRS-2, and PI-3 are not properly activated, which in turn prevents the normal kinase cascade from being triggered. The result is a malfunctioning cell, insulin resistance, and elevated levels of glucose and fatty acids within the blood.

This breakdown in signal transduction also affects the mitochondria (energy batteries) within the cells, especially those in the muscles and liver. In health, the mitochondria burn glucose and fatty acids. But when cell signaling breaks down, the mitochondria furnaces do not burn fat as effectively. That means that the fatty acids build up even more in the blood, and thus contribute to even greater insulin resistance. All of this results in an even greater overabundance of fuel in the bloodstream.

The brain recognizes this as dangerous, of course, and tells the pancreas to produce even more insulin. The pancreas does its best to produce more insulin, but the beta cells eventually wear out and can no longer meet the demands. At this point, the pancreas can no longer produce insulin.

Recovery

The key to restoring insulin sensitivity is to reduce the fatty acid content of the blood. A tripronged approach is best—weight loss, exercise, and a change in diet to include fewer processed foods, less fat, and more vegetables, whole grains, and fruit.

Weight loss alone can indeed restore insulin sensitivity. Weight loss reduces adipose tissue and fat reserves, which in turn reduce the fatty acid content of the blood. They also reduce the stresses placed on cells by cytokines and hormones.

Exercise also has the capacity to restore insulin sensitivity. As Dr. Wood points out, sumo wrestlers are often obese, but they are generally not insulin resistant. Exercise burns blood sugar and thus lowers insulin. It also forces the muscles and liver to burn glycogen and fatty acids, thus emptying the muscles and allowing them to serve as adequate storage tanks for glucose and glycogen when excess calories are consumed. Exercise also makes muscles more energy efficient. Muscle tissue is very active. Even while the body is largely at rest, muscles will burn more glucose than adipose tissue will. As muscles become larger from exercise, they serve as bigger storage tanks for glycogen. They also become more efficient at transforming glucose into glycogen, which means more fatty acids in the blood get safely stored and eventually burned.

Dietary change is also essential. Fewer processed foods mean fewer calories, which translates into weight loss, lower glucose, insulin, and triglyceride levels. Unprocessed foods, such as vegetables, whole grains, and fruit, are dense in nutrients and fiber and lower in calories, which promotes weight loss and balanced glucose and insulin levels. Furthermore, fiber-rich foods bind with insulin and help eliminate it from the body, thus lowering the overall insulin level.

All of these factors affect health in a multitude of ways, yet so much is in our personal control to take action and possibly reverse the damage.

Such advice is ageold. "About 800 years ago, Maimonides, a famous religious teacher and physician, taught not to overeat, and to eat slowly, and to not overeat fat," said Dr. Blackburn. "These ideas are still true today. They're part of our basic human wisdom. They keep us healthy, but we're not following them today and there are many serious consequences."

One of the biggest consequences to insulin imbalance, of course, is overweight, which is one of the greatest threats to health and life that we face today.

Healthy Blood Values

Blood glucose levels are measured in three different ways—a fasting test which is taken after a person has abstained from food for at least 12 hours; a two-hour postprandial test, in which a person has abstained from food for at least two hours; and a random test, taken any time without necessarily abstaining from food.

Healthy values for the three tests are as follows:

Fasting glucose test: between 70 and 99 mg/dl

Two hour postprandial test: between 70 and 145 mg/dl

Random test: between 70 and 125 mg/dl

A person is considered diabetic when his or her fasting glucose levels are 126 mg/dl, or higher, or his or her two-hour postprandial test glucose levels are 200 mg/dl or higher.

Blood cholesterol is divided into types, or fractions.

Low-density lipoprotein, or LDL cholesterol, is linked to heart disease and other serious illnesses.

High-density lipoprotein, or HDL cholesterol, protects the heart and arteries by taking LDL away from arteries and leading it to the liver, where it is neutralized and passed into the intestinal tract for elimination from the body. For this reason, HDL cholesterol is often referred to as the "good" cholesterol.

Total cholesterol is the number indicating the combined values of both HDL and LDL cholesterol.

The National Heart Lung and Blood Institute recommends that your LDL cholesterol should be lower than 100 milligrams per deciliter of blood (usually expressed as mg/dl). But many experts would like to see LDL fall below 80 or even 70.

The United States surgeon general recommends that HDL levels be 60 mg/dl or higher.

Ideally, totally cholesterol should fall around 150 mg/dl. Studies indicate that people with a blood cholesterol level at or around 150 mg/dl have extremely low rates of heart disease. Researchers point out that people with cholesterol levels above 180 mg/dl experience a sharp increase in the risk of heart disease and heart attack.

The surgeon general recommends that triglycerides, or blood fats, should be no higher than 150 mg/dl.

CHAPTER 5

Best Strategies for Overweight and Obesity

Plus size is the new normal

We read a lot about the numbers of people who are overweight or obese, but very little about how the growing waistline of Americans is changing attitudes and business. The truth is, everybody is adjusting to expanded girth. And in some cases, it's designed to make us feel better about ourselves, even as we gain more weight. Here are some examples.

We're making clothing bigger, but labeling them as smaller sizes. Today's size 10 dress was sold in the 1940s as a size 14. Nike's small sports bra used to fit a woman with a 33- to 35-inch bust line. Today, Nike's small sports bra is designed for a woman with a 35- to 37-inch bust.

Business at plus-size boutiques is booming. Lane Bryant plans to nearly double the number of its stores nationwide over the next five years. Catherine's Plus Sizes is not far behind. The Gap, Limited, and Target are all selling plus sizes to children now.

We're making the seats bigger. When the Boston Red Sox renovated Fenway Park, they made the seats four inches wider. They had to in order to accommodate the average fan. Seattle's Puget Sound ferries had to create more benches and bigger seats for riders. The old seats were too small and too many people had to stand.

We're making the needles longer. Doctors are now using longer needles to administer vaccines, medicines, and draw blood. The old standard needles were too short to fully penetrate the thicker layers of fat on the arms of Americans as well as many other population groups.

We're allowing more weight on aircraft. The Federal Aviation Administration ordered airlines to add another ten pounds per person to the approved passenger weights.

Yo-Yo dieting

More and more of us have given up hope of ever being at a healthy body weight again. The patient Robert was one such example.

He stood 5 feet 11 inches tall and weighed 290 pounds. He was morbidly obese, but that was only part of his trouble. His total blood cholesterol level was 280 mg/dl, which meant that he had galloping atherosclerosis in his coronary arteries. He had high blood pressure and painful bouts of claudication—leg pain caused by poor circulation. He was insulin resistant and taking oral medication for diabetes. He regularly suffered from shortness of breath and occasional arrhythmia, especially when he climbed stairs. His feet were so swollen and numb that he constantly feared infection and the loss of one or more of his toes.

Like so many overweight Americans, Robert was a chronic dieter—he'd tried them all—and although he did occasionally lose weight, he regularly gained back the lost pounds shortly after losing them. The problem was that he couldn't stay on a diet—they all represented some form of unendurable hunger to him. Truth be told, he didn't have much hope of ever succeeding on any weight loss plan until his doctor explained insulin to him.

More than calories

Robert thought that dieting was all about calories, which is partially true, but there is more to it than that. In simple terms, we gain weight when we eat more calories than we burn; we lose weight when we burn more calories than we eat. But this simple formula is actually too simplistic to help in creating a practical and effective weight loss program, especially for overweight people whose diets chronically fail them.

"Before I understood insulin," Robert recalled, "my diets were either austere, or loaded with fat. I was either on the high-carbohydrate, low-fat diet, which didn't give me any real pleasure, or I was on the high-protein, low-carb diet, which made me feel physically and mentally terrible.

I couldn't win. But when my doctor told me how insulin works, and I started reading about how insulin is related to weight, I began to understand how I could eat a low-calorie diet that allowed me to enjoy foods that made me feel satisfied and full, but at the same time caused me to lose weight. For example, I love pasta with vegetables cooked in olive oil. And I love to sauté my vegetables in olive or sesame oil. A diet based on the principle of low insulin allowed me to eat all of these foods, and lose weight at the same time."

In 14 months, Robert lost 100 pounds, and he has kept the weight off for more than two years. "I don't believe I will ever be fat again," he said recently. "I know how to keep my weight down now."

Robert is one of the lucky ones, and unfortunately part of a minority.

US and China rising obesity levels

Most Americans (two-thirds) are overweight, and half of those are obese. What's worse, the number of overweight and obese people is rising with frightening speed. About 30 years ago, only 15% of adult Americans were obese. Today that number has more than doubled (30.5%). In some cities in China the incidence is almost 20%, a dramatic change from times when China experienced famine.

Multiple problems

The problems associated with overweight and obesity go beyond the esthetics of physical appearance, though, when you consider the psychological impact of excess weight on children and adults. This is one of the reasons it has become a national issue. Children who are overweight are often ostracized and teased. Many grow up seeing themselves as fat, ugly, and unworthy of love—conditions that affect them their entire lives. Obese adults are confronted with situations every day in which their size places them in untenable or humiliating circumstances.

Then there are the health effects of overweight and obesity. Some of the diseases include heart disease, high blood pressure, stroke, diabetes, gallbladder disease, and possibly even a link to cancers. Today, the costs associated with obesity-related illnesses have reached $117 billion. Obesity may have just caught up to tobacco as a leading cause of death and disability.

Sedentary kids

Health experts are unanimous in their assertion that the underlying cause of overweight and obesity is poor diet and lack of exercise. Children today have more incentives to be sedentary than to be active. Even the staple of an after school sport has often fallen by the wayside. In the late 1960s, 80% of children participated in a sport on a daily basis. Today, only 20% do. Television, video games, the Internet, and continuous digital connectivity keep children sedentary. It's often the exception rather than the rule that kids get out after school to play basketball, soccer, tennis, football, or baseball with friends.

Food confusion and too much choice

And then there is the problem of food. Has any generation of humans ever been more confused about what to eat than our own? The plethora of food and diet experts—many of whom disagree with each other—only seems to make matters worse. Most Americans have tried and failed on a wide variety of diets. Why are we so clueless on a subject that was second nature to our grandparents and forebears?

Part of the problem with diets and dieting most certainly rests with the fact that we have so many food choices today. There is more food available to us than at any other time in human existence. Meanwhile, food manufacturers have created thousands of new foods that tantalize the taste buds but do not contribute to our health. Fast food may be convenient and tasty, but it makes us fat and sick. In the supermarket aisles, we must read labels, understand complicated, scientific terms, and try to determine if the foods we purchase will cause disease. Food has become complicated and dangerous, which is why so many of us turn to experts for help.

Which diet?

There is no limit to the number of advisors out there, and there are countless eating plans and proposed weight-loss programs. Essentially, two regimens have dominated in the last three decades—the low-fat, high-carbohydrate regimen, and the low-carbohydrate, high-protein diet.

Originally, the high-carbohydrate, low-fat regimen was composed largely of unprocessed foods, such as whole grains, fresh vegetables, beans, fruit, and low-fat animal products. All of these foods are low in calories and rich in nutrition. They also keep insulin levels relatively low. Not surprisingly, many people lost weight on this approach, and thousands more were able to reverse serious illnesses. But the restrictions of the low-fat, high-carb diet—especially when it comes to healthful fats such as olive, sesame, and safflower oils—make it unsatisfying for many.

Refined high GI carbohydrates

During the late 1980s and 1990s, the high-carb diet went through a strange metamorphosis that went largely unnoticed in the press. Food manufactures, responding to an enormous trend in the marketplace, began offering carbohydrate-rich foods that were highly processed and loaded with calories. They labeled these foods "Low Fat!" or "No Fat!" but they are nonetheless loaded with calories—rapidly absorbed calories (high glycemic index) which means they have a devastating effect on insulin levels, raising them through the roof. Thus, the once-healthy low-fat, high-carb diet soon became the high-carb, high-calorie, high-insulin diet, which is one of the primary reasons so many people of all ages are overweight today.

High protein

The almost predictable reaction to the failure of the low-fat diet was the high-protein diet, which was low in carbohydrates, but often rich in fat. That diet certainly facilitated much weight loss, but for many it was unsustainable, as it caused a wide variety of side effects, which for many people included constipation, headaches, bad breath, joint pain, and a constant craving for the body's primary source of fuel, carbohydrates. High-protein diets can also promote bone loss, osteoporosis, and kidney disorders, among other serious conditions.

Too much protein causes damage

Protein is converted in the body into acid, which is then eliminated from the blood by the kidneys. Your brain monitors your blood-acid levels—or pH—very carefully. It is continually attempting to maintain a balanced pH, or a slightly alkaline state. When blood acid-levels rise too high, the brain signals the bones to release phosphorus and calcium, which naturally alkalize the blood and restore its balanced pH. These minerals neutralize the excess acid, but at a price. The loss of calcium and phosphorus weakens bones. If this bone loss continues, your bones can eventually become porous and osteoporotic. High blood acidity also can weaken and eventually injure the kidneys, which are forced to eliminate as much acid from the blood as possible.

High-protein diets, of course, cause elevations in both protein and acid levels within the blood, which sets off a domino effect that can ultimately result in osteoporosis and kidney disease.

By 2016 it is apparent that, on the whole, both high-carbohydrate and high-protein diets have clearly failed. There are many people still clinging to the high-protein diet but undoubtedly, long term, it is unhealthy. Any weight loss achieved on either one was quickly gained back after people abandoned one or both approaches. At this point, most of us are confused, and a great many are cynical about the whole subject. Meanwhile, the epidemic of overweight and obesity only gets worse.

No hope?

This does not mean that weight loss and health promotion cannot be achieved. It only means that the two dominant approaches have been unable to satisfy both our palates and our concerns about weight and health.

It's worth remembering that our ancestors, no matter whether they came from—Europe, the Mediterranean region, Africa, or Asia—never thought about dieting. Yet, most were lean. Even today many populations, especially those in Asia and the Mediterranean, are still lean and experience relatively lower rates of the illnesses that we experience today.

Junk food

Processed foods are uniformly dangerous. From an insulin, calorie, and weight-loss standpoint, they are concentrated packages of calories that are rapidly absorbed, cause insulin to spike, and fat to be stored in the tissues. When fat is added to them, they're even worse. As we've discussed in previous chapters, insulin is a storage hormone.

Right now, as you read this book, your cells are hopefully utilizing a fuel mix that is composed of about 50% glucose and 50% fat. (So long as you are not munching on a pound of potato chips!) As long as your insulin level remains relatively low, you are burning a mixture of blood sugar and fat. But let's say that you eat a bagel, doughnut, or chocolate bar. Immediately, your blood is flooded with glucose. Your body sees this as an emergency situation and releases an abundance of insulin so that your cells will burn as much excess glucose as possible.

"Stop burning fat," says your brain!

In order to enhance glucose burning, your brain instructs your cells to stop burning fat—just burn sugar, and nothing else, it says. This will help to bring your glucose levels down into the safe ranges. Your body does this to keep you from going into a diabetic coma.

As we saw in the last chapter, the body usually cannot burn all the calories that are consumed, especially from processed foods. The excess blood sugar that cannot be burned must instead be converted to triglycerides (fatty acids) and stored in your tissues as fat.

Yum, a bag of potato chips!

All those excess calories in processed foods are not the only problem, however. Most processed foods also contain fat. So, let's say that rather than snacking on a bagel, which contains virtually no fat, you eat potato chips, which are rich in both processed carbs and fat. The carbohydrates in the potato chips go into the bloodstream and become glucose. The fat is also absorbed into your blood. Instantly, your body says, "Shut off fat burning and instead burn as much glucose as possible." At the same time, your body stores the fat from the potato chips in your tissues. In addition, any glucose that cannot be burned is also stored as fat in your tissues. Both the fat and the excess carbs become fat on your belly, buttocks, arms, shoulders, and legs.

Like most processed foods, potato chips are high in calories. A pound of potato chips provides about 2400 calories. The body needs approximately 10 calories to maintain 1 pound of body weight. That means that that 2,400 calories supports the weight of a 240-pound person. If you eat a pound of potato chips and you weigh less than 240 pounds, you're gaining weight. If you already weigh 240 pounds and you eat a pound of chips, you're also gaining weight because you are presumably eating more than just the chips that day. Which is why potato chips, like most processed foods, make us fat.

What about the good fats?

But here's an interesting fact that most of us don't understand: if you eat a mono- or polyunsaturated fat, such as olive oil, or sesame oil, or safflower oil with a low-calorie food, such as vegetables, you will actually promote weight loss, for two reasons. First, polyunsaturated fats tend to slow the rate at which carbohydrates are absorbed into the bloodstream. When cooked with olive oil, carbs tend to enter the bloodstream at a slower pace, which keeps insulin levels relatively low. When insulin levels are low, you keep burning fat that's stored in your tissues. Second, mono- and polyunsaturated fats stimulate your body to release stored fat into your bloodstream and burn it as fuel.

In order to understand how this happens, we must have a better understanding of the fat that we're carrying around on our bodies.

What is fat tissue?

The fat on our stomachs, buttocks, and elsewhere is known as adipose tissue. The cells that make up adipose tissue, called adipocytes, are capable of expanding up to 1,000 times their original size. Fat cells can get fat, which, of course, makes us fat.

The body stores fat as a backup fuel source. In fact, our ability to retain fat on our tissues was a form of adaptation that kept our early ancestors alive. As we will see in greater detail later on, people in ancient times—anywhere from 20,000 years ago to 400,000 years ago—who had relatively more fat on their tissues had a better chance of surviving food shortages, long migrations, and winters than those who were too lean. It seems that survival was not only for the fittest, but also for the fattest.

Two types of body fat

There are two forms of adipose tissue—one called visceral fat, which surrounds the internal organs, such as the kidneys, liver, spleen, and intestines, and the other called subcutaneous fat, which is found mostly around the buttocks and the belly.

Visceral fat is highly volatile and shed relatively easily. A little exercise and a reduction in calorie consumption cause this fat to be mobilized and rapidly burned as fuel. The body sees visceral fat as a ready and quick source of energy whenever it is needed. It's analogous to your basic candy bar. If you're playing basketball, or tennis, or out walking, you'll burn the fuel stored in your muscles. Once that's gone, your body will call on its visceral fat to meet its energy needs.

Subcutaneous fat, on the other hand, is much more intractable and stubborn, in large part because the body regards this form of fat as a long-term fuel supply, especially when food shortages endure. Consequently, the body is much more reluctant to surrender it, because it could be a life-saving form of energy when food is scarce. In modern life, of course, subcutaneous fat is that last ten pounds that are so difficult to shed.

Fat distribution in men vs. women

Men tend to have relatively more visceral fat, while premenopausal women relatively more subcutaneous fat. This makes sense from an evolutionary standpoint. Premenopausal women are capable of giving birth. Therefore, nature equipped them with more long-term energy supplies in the event of a pregnancy.

Men, who traditionally did more manual labor, need

a ready and accessible supply of energy when glycogen levels fall. Hence, the purpose of visceral fat—the quick pick-me-up fat that is stored around your organs and deep inside your belly and can be rapidly mobilized and burned when instant energy is needed.

A storage depot or a hive of activity?

Scientists used to believe that adipose tissue—whether it was visceral or subcutaneous—was nothing more than a storage depot for energy. They also thought that fat was highly inactive—everyone believed that it remained inactive, and waited for the moment when it was needed. But recent discoveries have changed these notions.

Adipose tissue, it turns out, is now recognized as an endocrine organ, meaning an organ that produces hormones. Not only is it highly active, but it is also essential for the healthy functioning of the entire body. Adipocytes produce an array of hormones that act as messengers to the entire system. Among them are tumor necrosis factor, which in small amounts is good but, when produced in excess, can lead to inflammation and heart disease. They also produce estrogen, the female sex hormone, and a substance called leptin.

Leptin: one of the keys to understanding fat gain

Leptin, from the Greek word *leptos*, which means "thin," regulates appetite and food intake as well as glucose and fat burning. When the body has stored enough energy as fat, adipose tissues increase the production of leptin, which sends a signal to an organ in the brain called the hypothalamus. The hypothalamus, in turn, sends out a signal to the brain and stomach to stop eating, lose appetite, and recognize that you are now satiated. The hypothalamus also signals muscles throughout the body to start burning excess fat stored in the muscles and other tissues. Scientists have identified an enzyme or kinase within the hypothalamus called AMPK (activated protein kinase), which signals the hypothalamus to send out the message to stop eating and start burning fat.

At the same time, the burst of leptin tells skeletal muscles throughout the body—again, by stimulating AMPK—to burn glucose and fat supplies in the muscles. That will lower weight all by itself. But when the muscles empty their energy supplies, they become good storage tanks for excess glucose and fat for the next time we eat a processed or high-fat food. When the body can store excess glucose and fat, it does not have such high levels of glucose in the blood, which means that it does not have to produce so much insulin. One of the benefits of low insulin is that the body will keep on burning fat as part of its fuel mix.

Thus, under healthy conditions, leptin lowers your appetite, limits your food intake, and keeps you burning both fat and glucose. Leptin also increases insulin sensitivity, which means you need less insulin to do the same job—another way leptin keeps insulin levels low, and fat burning high.

Leptin resistance

When scientists first discovered leptin in 1994, they immediately thought that they had found the answer to overweight and obesity. Give people more leptin, they reasoned, and they will immediately eat less and burn more fat. Alas, that was not the case. In fact, leptin levels were already higher in obese individuals, researchers soon discovered. And when obese people were given leptin therapeutically, they did not respond as expected. The hypothalamus, the major site of leptin signaling, failed to react to the increase in leptin signaling. As it turned out, the hypothalamus and muscles in overweight and obese people had become resistant to leptin's instructions. Later studies showed that the gene that, under normal circumstances, would otherwise respond to leptin, failed to react to the leptin signaling. Consequently, the hypothalamus did not send out a message to the body stop eating and start burning fat.

Laboratory studies found that obese mice have higher-than-normal leptin levels, but that they nonetheless sit under the food hopper and continue to eat. They remain hungry long after their stomachs are full and their bodies require no more energy. People respond in similar ways, later studies discovered. Sami T Azar in the *American Journal of Medical Sciences*, April 2002, demonstrates that obese people have higher-than-normal leptin levels. The leptin simply fails to do its job.

Interestingly, even in overweight and obese people, leptin works for a time, but its messages are eventually overridden and fail. The disorder that arises when leptin no longer makes us feel full, and fails to stimulate fat burning, is called *leptin resistance.*

What makes us leptin resistant or sensitive?

Later studies showed that leptin resistance arises with the elevation of a specific protein, known as PTP1B, which blocks leptin signaling within the cells of the hypothalamus. What increases this pernicious protein? Saturated fat from red meat and dairy products. Researchers found that as saturated fat intake increases, so too does PTP1B, which in turn makes the hypothalamus and muscle tissue resistant to leptin.

Saturated fats make us eat more, in part, because they weaken leptin's impact on our appetite.

On the other hand, vegetable oils—specifically mono-unsaturated and polyunsaturated fats—restore leptin sensitivity and effectiveness. Numerous studies have shown that fish oils, polyunsaturated omega-3 fats, perform the remarkable feat of restoring leptin sensitivity and insulin sensitivity as well as promoting fat burning.

Switch your fats!

For anyone who is overweight, diabetic, or insulin resistant, a switch from saturated fat to mono- and polyunsaturated fats is an essential step. You will very likely have more control over your appetite, eat less, feel satisfied, and lose weight faster if you eat moderate amounts of polyunsaturated and monounsaturated fats than if you eat saturated fats from beef and dairy products.

Moreover, whole, unprocessed plant foods are nutrient-rich, low-fat foods. When low-calorie plant foods are combined with moderate amounts of olive, sesame, or safflower oil, as well as with low-calorie animal foods, you arrive at a diet that is both low in calories and highly satisfying. In addition, it will keep insulin levels low, which means you will continue to burn fat.

Moderate amounts of oil are a tablespoon of olive, sesame, or safflower oil, which contains approximately 250 calories. For people who want to lose weight, a tablespoon can be used several times a week or even daily, depending on how much weight you want to lose, and how fast you want to do it. The oil can be added to cooking, or added to raw vegetables. The Mediterranean diet is just one example of how traditional people—the French, Italians, Greeks, Israelis, and North Africans—use precisely this combination of vegetables, low-fat animal products, and oils to create a diet that is low in calories and rich in nutrition. The Mediterranean diet, as you know, is associated with low rates of all the modern illnesses, including heart disease, the common cancers, diabetes, Alzheimer's, and Parkinson's disease.

Red wine!

Interestingly, one more substance also increases leptin sensitivity—a substance in red wine, known as resveratrol, acts as a PTP1B blocker and thus restores leptin sensitivity to the hypothalamus and to muscle tissue. Scientists speculated that resveratrol could be one of the keys to the well-known "French paradox"—the term frequently used to describe the fact that the French people, who drink moderate amounts of red wine and eat plenty of fatty foods, are nonetheless lean. The French have relatively low rates of obesity and overweight, especially when compared to Americans.

Exercise

It is almost too good to be true. Yet it is true. Exercise has demonstrated the most remarkable benefits on all body and brain pathways. Interestingly, researchers have found that exercise, even a 20-minute walk per day, causes a very similar effect as leptin on the brain, muscles, appetite, fat burning, and insulin levels. In fact, exercise triggers the same kind of signal transduction as leptin on skeletal muscles. Once we begin walking, AMPK is triggered, signaling muscles to burn fat and glycogen stores. At the same time, exercise increases insulin sensitivity. Both of these alterations in biochemistry results in some weight loss and, more importantly, lower insulin levels.

These same effects have been found in people all ages, even the elderly. Researchers at Case Western Reserve University School of Medicine in Cleveland, Ohio, examined 16 obese men, all of them 63 years of age or older, who walked on a treadmill and/or road a cycle machine daily. All of them were insulin resistant at the start of the study. No changes in diet were made, but after 12 weeks of walking or cycling, all had lost weight and had overcome insulin resistance. (Halberg N, Erikson M et al., *Journal of Applied Physiology*, December 22, 2005.)

Exercise burns calories, of course, but that is not the primary way that it causes weight loss. A three-mile walk or run might only burn 350 calories, and you'd need to do 10 such walks in order to lose a single pound of body weight (the equivalent of 3,500 calories). Fortunately, this is only one way that exercise contributes to weight loss, and perhaps the least efficient way. Exercise builds muscle mass, which is highly active tissue that is constantly burning higher levels of fat, even when you are not exercising. It also improves the efficiency of muscles, increasing fat burning. When muscles are exercised, their glycogen stores are emptied, freeing them up to take on excess glucose. This means that when glucose levels become elevated—after eating a processed food, for example—the body can place more glucose in the muscle tissue and thus maintain lower insulin levels. With lower insulin, more fat is burned, even while you are resting. All of this contributes to weight loss.

Reversing insulin resistance

With regular exercise, we can essentially reverse insulin resistance.

Exercise physiologists point out that, while a daily, 30-minute exercise routine should be the goal, we can accomplish nearly as much with three 10-minute walks per day. Such a program can be greatly enhanced by engaging in an hour of exercise on the weekends, such as walking, either outside or on a treadmill, or riding an indoor cycle machine, or playing a game that you enjoy. Such an exercise program can give us all the physiological and health-restoring benefits described here. When these movements are coupled with a low-calorie, high-nutrient, high-satiety diet, even obesity can be overcome.

Food is addictive

Nora Volkow, director of the National Institute of Drug Abuse, has shown that food and illicit drugs share the same reward circuitry in the brain. Both increase the neurotransmitter known as dopamine. Dopamine, in turn, triggers the reward centers of the brain, which means that both food and drugs make us feel good. And, not surprisingly, both can be addictive.

Researchers hypothesize that low dopamine levels may trigger food cravings, even when one is not otherwise hungry for food. Interestingly, scientists have also found that normal insulin signaling in the brain stimulates the release of dopamine. That means that normal insulin function may result in higher dopamine, more consistent states of well-being—thanks to the well-stimulated reward centers—and low food cravings. That very sequence could explain why many people are not overcome by food cravings and find it easy to maintain normal body weight.

On the other hand, people with insulin resistance experience a decrease in dopamine signaling, which in turn stimulates food cravings. Eating elevates dopamine and alleviates the food cravings, at least temporarily. But as dopamine falls, cravings rise, even when food consumption is harmful.

Findings like these are behind the search for new ways to elevate dopamine and stimulate the brain's reward centers, without turning to food. At the Sackler School of Medicine at Tel Aviv University in Israel, Dr. Tviv Barak is using a pharmaceutical drug containing histamine in order to signal the brain that the person has consumed enough food and now feels full and satisfied. Histamine is a naturally occurring neurotransmitter in that it's already present in the brain. When histamine binds with certain receptors in the brain, known as H-1 receptors, people experience a decrease in appetite and an increase in fullness and satisfaction from food.

Serotonin

Meanwhile, researchers are using other chemical neurotransmitters in the brain in order to stimulate higher levels of satisfaction with smaller quantities of food. One approach is to increase brain levels of serotonin, the neurotransmitter responsible for feelings of well-being, safety, relaxation, and contentment. Researchers have noticed that when depressed people are placed on serotonin uptake inhibitors—such as Prozac—they experience a decrease in appetite and lose weight. Brain levels of serotonin are boosted after we eat a meal that contains carbohydrates. Carbohydrate-rich foods increase blood levels of an amino acid called tryptophan, which in turn increases brain levels of serotonin. Researchers are attempting to use low-calorie, high-carbohydrate diets to increase brain levels of serotonin, which they hope will decrease appetite, increase satisfaction from food, and bring about weight loss.

Gorging and bingeing

In a very real sense, we are designed to accumulate and conserve calories. Our Paleolithic ancestors experienced extreme fluctuations in their food supply, which meant that whenever a large meal presented itself, they gorged on it. Gorging became an essential survival strategy, says Kerin O'Dea, PhD, in her article "Obesity and Diabetes in the 'Land of Milk and Honey'" (*Diabetes/Metabolism Reviews,* 1992). Our ancestors never knew for certain when their next meal might come, of if it would be adequate to keep them alive.

Gorging, of course, means taking in as much nutrition and calories as possible in a single meal. Most of the food that was available to our ancestors were plant foods, such as roots, tubers, stems, leafy vegetables, and fruit. We supplemented these foods with wild game, which provided fat, the single greatest source of calories in the food supply. The fact is, however, that there wasn't much fat to go around. In their seminal study entitled "Paleolithic Nutrition," researchers S. Boyd Eaton, MD, and Melvin Konner, PhD (*New England Journal of Medicine,* 1985), report that, unlike today's fatted livestock, the average animal killed and eaten by our Paleolithic forebears was extremely lean. They were probably no different than animals living today in Africa, which Konner and Eaton report have only 3.9%

body fat. The total calories derived from fat from such an animal is no more than 20–25%, which meant that there wasn't a lot of fat on the animals our forebears ate. (Compare that to today's average hamburger, which derives 50% of its calories from fat.)

Not only were the animals lean, but they also weren't exactly easy to catch. Remember that we were not the greatest hunters in the early part of our existence. It wasn't until some 50,000 years ago that *homo habilis*, designated by anthropologists as "the toolmaker," emerged. Before that, we very likely had to track and run down small game, or get larger animals to fall into deep crevices where they would be killed.

Dr. A. S. Truswell of the Department of Nutrition and Food Science at the University of London has studied the !Kung of Botswana, a people who have maintained their traditional ways of living and eating since Paleolithic times. Truswell points out that it takes the !Kung women four hours to gather 1,000 calories of plant foods from the forest. On the other hand, it takes the men ten hours to capture the calorie equivalent in fresh game meat.

Genetic disposition: an instinct to overeat!!

Over time, we developed a genetic predisposition to eat as much as possible, whenever possible—a behavior Robert Pritikin, in his book, *The Pritikin Weight Loss Breakthrough* (Dutton Books, 1998), has termed "the fat instinct." Over the millennium, nature equipped us with a genetic drive to eat as much food as possible, whenever it was presented to us—and to instinctively choose fat in order to maximize our calorie intake.

Of course, during ancient times, nature herself protected us from diseases of overnutrition by limiting the food supply, and the amount of fat we could obtain. Nature gave us an abundance of low-calorie plant foods, and supplemented them with animal foods, which were low in fat. That, in all probability, was the diet we evolved on, and the one we are still best suited to consume.

The problem we face today is that nature no longer controls the food supply. At least in the West, and at this moment in history, farming has triumphed over the vicissitudes of nature. The result is an abundance of food, a great percentage of which is loaded with fat and, thanks to food processing, packed with calories.

The great accomplishments of modern humans—our ability to create an abundant food supply and our increasing release from manual labor—is, to a great degree, working against our genetic design. Although we cannot go back in time, we must, in a certain sense, recreate the eating patterns of our ancestors if we are to restore our health and survive as a species. That means eating far more whole, unprocessed plant foods and limiting the quantities of animal foods, especially those rich in saturated fat. At the same time, we must increase our physical activity. To our ancestors, daily life was an enormous physical struggle simply to stay alive. For us, physical activity must be conscious forms of exercise.

As the following chapters of this book reveal, virtually all of the illnesses that we face today, especially those that are having the most widespread and devastating effects on our health, arise from lifestyles that are in conflict with our basic genetic design. As science delves ever deeper into the human genome, and we discover more about the mysterious workings of our cells, we learn that health is founded on a clear and fairly intractable set of behaviors. When we run afoul of those behaviors, we suffer the consequences. The good news is that even after we become ill, those same behaviors, like a powerful form of medicine, can restore us to health.

CHAPTER 6

Mending the Heart

A "fire within"

As toxic and as dangerous as insulin resistance is, it rarely if ever appears alone. Much more common is for it to appear with its standard accomplice, inflammation.

In truth, inflammation usually arises first. As the condition worsens, it forms the foundation for its Siamese twin, insulin resistance. Together they form the basis for an array of serious illnesses, including heart disease, cancer, diabetes, and Alzheimer's disease.

As discussed in chapter 1, in the strictest sense, inflammation is nothing more than the immune system's assault on a threat to your health. Coined by the ancient Greeks to mean "a fire within," the term inflammation describes the outward symptoms of that assault—heat, fever, redness, and swelling. Some or all of these symptoms emerge when your immune system is busy attacking a disease-causing agent, such as a bacteria or virus. That attack is an altogether good thing. In fact, it's one of the reasons we have survived as a species. But like any attack, we don't want it to go on for too long.

Under healthy conditions, the immune system's reaction to any given threat is ferocious, effective, and relatively short lived. The immune system is designed to identify the problem, destroy it, and then stand down, thus resuming a state of cool quiescence. Unfortunately, that doesn't happen for most of us.

Collateral damage

The problem today is that our blood, organs, lymph system, and joints are so filled with toxic substances that our immune systems are constantly attacking a multitude of dastardly invaders. If our immune systems could talk, they would tell us that there are just too many battles to fight. As in any war zone, there's significant collateral damage. The system is attacking the bad guys, but during those attacks, it can deform or destroy otherwise healthy tissue.

Inflammation and vessel plaque

One such example occurs when your immune system attacks the LDL cholesterol particles that infiltrate the tissues of your arteries. Immune cells attempt to destroy the LDL particles, but in the process cause the artery tissue to become swollen and filled with atherosclerotic plaques that can lead to a heart attack and stroke.

Inflammation occurs in tissues throughout the body. When it occurs in the brain, it can lead dementia and Alzheimer's disease. Elsewhere, it can lead to colon, breast, and prostate cancers, as well as diabetes, rheumatoid arthritis, diabetes, asthma, glaucoma, kidney disease, blindness, and many other serious disorders.

The root of most disease

The realization that the immune system plays a pivotal role in the onset of most degenerative diseases has given scientists new insights into today's major killers. For years, scientists knew that people with rheumatoid arthritis and even gingivitis had higher rates of heart disease, even when their cholesterol levels were normal. They also knew that people with diabetes had higher rates of Alzheimer's. "What possibly could be the connection between gingivitis and heart disease?" physicians asked. "Or, for that matter, diabetes and Alzheimer's?" That link is their common root—inflammation, which can deform joints and swell gums, and at the same time destroy arteries and brain tissue.

The most widespread of those conditions, of course, is cardiovascular disease, or illnesses of the heart and arteries, as well as strokes (and their aftereffects), which currently afflict approximately 85 million Americans, and kills close to 1 million of us each year. This is a staggering problem; for example, 230 million Chinese people have some form of cardiovascular disease. Heart disease has been the number one killer since 1900 (the sole exception was in 1918, when influenza and pneumonia topped the charts). Heart disease kills an American every 34 seconds, and 2,500 of us each day.

Grim as these statistics may be, they're going to get worse. More than 1 million American teenagers have metabolic syndrome (see chapter 4), a primary risk factor for heart disease.

Metabolic Syndrome is defined by the following characteristics:

1. Abdominal obesity or increased weight circumference
2. Elevated triglycerides and low HDL cholesterol
3. Elevated blood pressure
4. Elevated inflammatory markers, such as C-reactive protein and LDL cholesterol

The word "emergency" doesn't come close to describing what we will face, both in terms of the sheer suffering, as well as the out-of-control health care costs that illness is causing.

This is where we must begin our investigation—to learn how inflammation and insulin resistance combine to create the most deadly illnesses affecting us today, and how they can be prevented and overcome.

Slow and tasty suicide

At Columbia University College of Physicians and Surgeons

in New York City, Mehmet Oz, MD, famed professor of surgery, author, and television personality, has seen pretty much everything there is to see on the inside of the human body. He is particularly knowledgeable about the workings of the heart and arteries, serving as director of the Cardiovascular Institute at Columbia University Medical Center. Dr. Oz put the story of heart disease succinctly: "To understand heart disease, you've got to understand inflammation first, and insulin resistance second," he said. "Inflammation is really the destruction of the body by friendly fire. Our own immune system is turned against us, which is pretty scary when you realize just how powerful that system is."

The irony is that we are the ones turning that system against ourselves. We do it with behaviors that so many of us think nothing of, like eating a few hamburgers each week, piling on some French fries, and topping them off with some rich desserts.

Bad cholesterol

Hamburgers and French fries—not to mention many desserts—are loaded with saturated fat, which raises the bad cholesterol in your blood, the type known as LDL, or low-density lipoprotein. Once these foods, and others like them, are consumed, particles of LDL come flying into your bloodstream and migrate into your artery walls. In small amounts, those LDL particles would pass safely in and out of the artery tissue. But when LDL becomes elevated in your blood, those particles enter your artery walls and get stuck inside, like too many fat men trying to get out of a single doorway at the same time. The LDL piles up inside the artery tissue and then undergoes a most unfortunate change—it becomes oxidized.

Oxidation: "the rusting of arteries"

Simply put, oxidation is decay. The molecules inside the LDL break up, lose electrons, and become unstable, forming new chemical arrangements that kill or deform cells, tissues, and organs. Oxidation is the process that makes skin wrinkle, organs shrink, milk sour, apples brown, and iron rust. It is what most of us call aging.

In the body, oxidation can turn healthy cells and tissues into nonfunctioning scar tissue, or cholesterol plaques, or even cancer cells and tumors. It's something like the invasion of the body snatchers, in which healthy cells are turned into destructive ones.

Your immune system recognizes the problem and realizes that it's got to do something about it.

"The body is binary," said Dr. Oz. "It's either quiescent or inflamed. If the immune system senses that something bad is happening, it sends out the storm troopers, which are macrophage cells, to take it out." And that's where inflammation starts.

Macrophages and CD4 cells

Macrophages are very powerful immune cells that are sent into the artery walls, where they start gobbling up the decaying LDL particles. Unfortunately, once they've got the LDL inside their stomachs, the macrophages become bloated, poisoned, and eventually die.

Once the macrophages are neutralized, they too accumulate inside the walls of the artery. Before they die, they send out an SOS message to the rest of the immune system. They do this by producing cytokines, chemical messengers that contact the immune system's generals, which are called CD4 cells. "Send in reinforcements," the macrophages signal. "There's too much LDL here." Thanks to the cytokines, more macrophages arrive, eat the LDL, get sick, and accumulate inside the artery wall, causing the artery to become swollen and hard. This robs the artery of its normal flexibility, preventing it from expanding when the body needs to send more blood to the heart and other organs.

Complicating the problem is the fact that macrophages release oxidants as a way to kill disease-causing invaders, such as bacteria or viruses. In this setting, however, the release of oxidants only backfires—they promote the decay of LDL particles in the artery, which means that more immune cells must be called to the battle zone. There, the macrophages engorge more LDL and are poisoned and destroyed.

"Inflammation is the rusting of your arteries," said Dr. Oz succinctly. As tissue that needs to be flexible and capable of rapid expansion, arteries cannot afford to rust.

Hardened arteries—no expanding

So let's say that you climb a flight of stairs, or suddenly

experience stress. The heart immediately starts pumping more blood into the system. Under normal circumstances, the arteries would suddenly dilate to allow more blood to flow to the cells and the heart itself. Unfortunately, the hardened arteries cannot expand as extensively as they formerly could. With increased blood flow comes more pressure within the arterial system. It's not unlike squeezing a garden hose while the water is running.

Cracks in the vessels

As pressure within the artery increases, tiny cracks and fissures break open inside the inner linings of the arteries. This same cracking and fissuring can occur elsewhere, such as the kidneys or eyes, thus damaging these organs as well. When the pressure becomes great enough, arteries can burst open. If that happens in the brain, a stroke occurs. If it takes place in the heart, a heart attack can ensue.

But even if an artery doesn't rupture, it still has open wounds that are exposed to infiltration by decaying LDL particles and attacking immune cells—both of which combine to create more inflammation in the artery wall.

We continue eating those hamburgers, fried chicken, fatty desserts, or nachos and cheese, all of which are rich in saturated fat. That means that the LDL particles keep coming, and the macrophages keep eating the poison.

Formation of foam cells

Once they've become engorged with LDL, the macrophages

are called "foam cells"—they are literally foamy with LDL bloating. Eventually, they become so numerous that they break through the tile-like inner lining of the artery wall, called the *endothelial layer*, which is where the blood flows, forming a fatty streak.

Homocysteine is a corrosive agent

"The problem is made worse when homocysteine shows up and acts like acid on that endothelial layer," Dr. Oz pointed out.

Homocysteine is a highly corrosive amino acid that reaches dangerous levels when we eat too much red meat, dairy products, eggs, and chicken—in short, animal proteins. These proteins elevate methionine levels, which are converted into homocysteine, an amino acid that acts like acid rain on the delicate endothelial tissue.

"The inside lining of the artery is like Teflon," said Dr. Oz. "It creates a smooth surface so that blood can easily pass through the artery. Homocysteine burns away some of that surface to expose the medial layer below the Teflon coating. Once it's exposed, it attracts more LDL particles and immune cells. That medial layer is electrically charged. So the result is something like a thunderstorm inside your arteries."

A wound in the artery

Your body responds to a wound inside your artery wall in much the same way as it does to a wound anywhere else in the body. The liver is ordered via chemical messengers to produce clotting proteins that combine with blood platelets to form a Band-Aid over the open wound. In order for that Band-Aid to be created, clotting proteins chemically join to form a sticky substance called *fibrinogen,* which is a kind of glue that binds platelets together. The sticky platelets form a scab over the wound and thus begin the healing process.

Sticky blood

Unfortunately for too many of us today, the liver overproduces clotting proteins, which in turn make too much fibrinogen. These cause the blood to become sticky, which in turn causes platelets to clump together and form clots within the blood. Those blood clots can be big enough to reduce the flow of blood to the heart, brain, or other organs. They can also break free from the wound in the artery, float downstream, and get lodged in a smaller vessel, where it can block blood flow entirely to a vital organ.

Lifestyle choices

There are numerous reasons why the liver overproduces fibrinogen, and most of them are related to lifestyle choices. One of the big ones, of course, is cigarette smoking, which causes drastic changes in the liver, which responds by producing higher levels of fibrinogen, which increases the likelihood of blood clots. Others include a lack of exercise, too much homocysteine in the blood, and chronic infections, including such seemingly benign conditions as gingivitis. Still another is the consumption of a high-fat diet. Recently, scientists found that hormone replacement therapy (HRT) also elevates fibrinogen. This may well be the reason why HRT is associated with a greater risk of heart attack in some women.

Contrary to what many believe, heart disease is the number one killer of women (many assume it's breast cancer). More than 9 million women suffer from coronary heart disease and each year 50,000 women die of the illness (compared to the 40,500 who die from breast cancer).

All of us can reduce fibrinogen levels—and inflammation overall—with daily exercise, cessation of smoking (if you do smoke), and a reduction in animal protein and saturated fats.

What is atherosclerosis?

One of the problems with poor lifestyle choices is that they are consistent—we tend to eat the same foods each day and engage in the same level of activity, or the lack of it. Consequently, LDL continues to pour into the blood, which means foam cells continue to accumulate inside the artery. Eventually they form a fatty streak, which, if the conditions go unchanged, will grow into full-blown plaque, a condition known as *atherosclerosis*.

Inside the plaque, tiny puddles of cholesterol lie in the bellies of the macrophages. Eventually, the stomachs of the macrophages burst open and release that cholesterol. Over time, the tiny puddles form larger pools of cholesterol inside the plaque. As they do, they make the plaque unstable and force it to eventually erupt, much like a boil. It spews forth its inner contents into the bloodstream and leaves behind a wound in the artery wall.

The body responds to this latest wound by sending more fibrinogen and blood platelets. But now the conditions are ripe for a much more dangerous event. The plaque is larger; there's more fibrinogen; the blood platelets are stickier, and prone to forming an even larger clot. A large clot can not only block the artery entirely, but it can also—more likely—break free, float downstream, and block blood flow to the heart or brain, thus causing a heart attack or stroke.

Interestingly, the National Heart Lung and Blood Institute—the cardiovascular wing of the National Institutes of Health—has reported that most heart attacks occur in people with relatively small plaques that block only 30% or less of the artery. That means that it isn't the size of the plaque that's so dangerous, but the plaque's tendency to rupture, along with the blood's tendency to form large clots. It's the clots that block blood flow to the heart and bring on a heart attack.

As if all of this were not bad enough, insulin resistance actually makes it worse.

Eric Topol, MD, is one of the giants of modern medicine. He is chairman of the Department of Cardiovascular Medicine and Genetics at Case Western Reserve University, and the chief academic officer and chairman of the Department of Cardiovascular Medicine at the Cleveland Clinic. He has more than 1,100 scientific publications and he's authored and edited 30 books, including the *Textbook of Interventional Cardiology*. Topol is soft spoken, friendly, and open. Physically lean and precise with his words, he nonetheless seemed utterly relaxed in conversation and even enjoyed going over the basic science that explains how we find ourselves in the current health crisis.

"There isn't any question that insulin resistance is epidemic and contributes to heart disease," he began, "in part because obesity rates are climbing. Overweight and obesity take people over the edge and cause a breakdown in many different areas of the body, including the function and health of the heart and arteries."

Insulin resistance and inflammation are joined in our fat tissue, says Dr. Topol. The more your insulin levels rise, and stay high, the more overweight you become.

Fatty tissue is an active organ

Adipose tissue is a highly active organ producing an array of inflammatory cytokines, including tumor necrosis factor (TNF) and interleukin-6 (IL-6). When secreted in higher-than-normal quantities, these chemicals degrade cells and tissues, most likely by oxidizing fat cells. Tumor necrosis factor alone degrades the membranes of cells throughout the body and increases the risk of insulin resistance. Studies have shown that TNF plays a central role in the onset of diabetes. Virtually everyone who is overweight has higher levels of TNF in their bloodstream.

Whenever a person is in insulin resistance, they're unable to burn all the glucose in their bloodstream. Forced to get rid of the excess blood sugar, the body converts it to fat and stores it as adipose tissue. That means that if you're insulin resistant, you're making more fat, and if you're making more fat, you're making more TNF and IL-6.

When cells are attacked by these inflammatory cytokines, the body calls out the macrophages to help eliminate the deformed cells and the high levels of TNF and IL-6. Once macrophages show up on the scene, however, they release more oxidants, which cause even greater damage and higher levels of inflammation.

TNF and IL-6 do not simply stay in the fatty tissue, however. They flow into the bloodstream and make their way to the main arteries, including the coronary arteries that lead to the heart. There they degrade artery tissue and add to the inflammation that's already taking place.

Sticky molecules: the body's Velcro

At that point, another group of cells arrive on the scene—these are called *adhesion molecules*. For a long time, scientists believed that these molecules were essentially the glue that held together ligaments, muscles, and just about everything else in the body. That alone is a pretty important job, but recent research has revealed that these tiny chemicals are involved in a lot of other activities as well, including directing the immune system's efforts to heal wounds, including wounds that occur in the arteries.

"Adhesion molecules are already present because the artery has been wounded by several factors, including by homocysteine and high blood pressure," said Dr. Topol. "They're already trying to repair the endothelium."

Adhesion molecules are the body's Velcro. They're

sticky. Once inside the artery, they start gluing all the chemical players together—TNF, IL-6, LDL, homocysteine, macrophages, platelets—you name it. That means that all of these highly inflammable substances are stuck inside the artery tissue, like a big crowd in an elevator. Something's got to give—and that something is often the artery wall itself. An even bigger, bulging plaque emerges, one that protrudes into the inner pathway of the artery. Moreover, these conditions, which only escalate, make the plaque more volatile and prone to rupture. The more rupturing of plaque occurs, the more at risk you are of creating a large clot that can trigger a heart attack or stroke.

Adiponectin, coming to the rescue

At this point, things may look pretty grim, but the body is nonetheless capable of producing substances that can come to the rescue. One of the most important of these is *adiponectin*.

Adiponectin is an anti-inflammatory hormone that can restore insulin sensitivity, and get all of those crowded cells, LDL, and cytokines out of the elevator. Once it arrives on the scene of the wound, adiponectin immediately sends out cytokines that communicate with all the many chemical and cellular players that are combining to cause the damage. Acting as a kind of traffic cop, the adiponectin orders the body to produce fewer adhesion molecules, thus allowing more of the inflammatory chemicals to pass freely from the site. It also cools the effects of the macrophages by suppressing their tendency to consume the TNC and other inflammatory chemicals in the area. Adiponectin also induces apoptosis in some cells that may cause additional problems in the healing of the artery wall. And finally, it increases insulin sensitivity. In fact, it is so good at this job that some studies have shown that high levels of adiponectin alone are enough to take a people out of insulin resistance.

There's a catch, however. The body can only produce adiponectin from lean adipocytes—or small fat cells. In other words, you've got to be at a normal or healthy weight to produce sufficient quantities of adiponectin to take you out of insulin resistance. People who are overweight or obese produce lower amounts of adiponectin, and more TNF and IL-6, which is one possible explanation why people with insulin resistance and hyperinsulinemia do not heal as quickly as those who are not insulin resistant.

The good news is that as people lose weight, their adiponectin production increases, which in turn provides all the positive effects of this powerful hormone. Meanwhile, scientists are researching ways to create new drugs that will increase adiponectin levels in insulin-resistant people, and thus decrease risk of heart disease. Adiponectin may be a powerful protector against cancer, as well.

Good cholesterol

Yet another safeguard in the body's fight against heart disease is HDL cholesterol, or high-density lipoprotein, otherwise known as the good cholesterol. HDL has exactly the opposite effect on arteries as LDL. Rather than bring cholesterol into the artery wall, HDL shepherds it away from the artery and over to the liver, where it is converted to a water-soluble substance and eliminated from the body through the feces.

HDL also acts as an antioxidant, preventing the decay of LDL and thus slowing the atherosclerotic process.

Fiber

Fiber also assists in the process by binding with fats, including saturated fats, in the gut and then eliminating them from the body. The more fiber in the diet, the less saturated fat goes into the liver. That means less LDL goes into the bloodstream.

The National Heart Lung and Blood Institute (NHLBI) urges people to adopt a diet and lifestyle that will keep LDL levels below 100 mg/dl. But Dr. Topol says that that number should go even lower.

"There are societies in Asia and Africa that have LDL levels below 70 mg/dl," said Dr. Topol. "And they don't suffer heart attacks. So I think that LDL number of 100 is a little high to feel safe. I'd like to see it at 70 or lower. In fact, we really haven't seen the LDL number be too low at this point."

As for HDL, the NHLBI recommends 60 mg/dl or higher. In the past, the US surgeon general recommended an HDL level of 40, but recent government agencies have urged people to go even higher.

Tips to reduce inflammation and raise HDL

1. Eat antioxidant-rich whole grains, vegetables, and fruits.
2. Antioxidant-rich food boosts your HDL, but it will bind with saturated fats and lower your LDL.
3. Eat niacin-rich foods, which include salmon, trout, nuts, beans, leafy greens, the white meat of chicken, the white meat of turkey, and peanut butter. Ask your doctor to monitor any use of niacin supplements, because they can be harmful to some people at even moderate doses.
4. Avoid sugar and other processed foods, which increase fat accumulation, insulin resistance, and lower HDL.
5. Eat a moderate amount of soy foods, such as soybeans, tofu, tempeh, miso, tamari, and shoyu. Soy foods may reduce LDL and triglycerides, while boosting HDL. (Excessive amounts of soya are not recommended as they do have an effect similar as estrogen on cells.)
6. Exercise daily. A 30–40 minute walk, or any other form of aerobic exercise, can significantly boost your HDL.
7. Lose body fat. As we've already seen, excess weight increases triglycerides and LDL, while lowering HDL. Conversely, weight loss boosts HDL levels.
8. Drink alcohol in moderation. Studies have shown that moderate amounts of alcohol (one to two drinks per day) can increase HDL, especially

if it is drunk during a meal. Some research suggests that alcohol consumed during a meal may move cholesterol deposits out of the artery wall.

9. Stop smoking.

10. Eat cooked grains that contain soluble fiber, such as oatmeal, brown rice, apples, grapes, and citrus fruits. These foods lower LDL and, after regular consumption for approximately three months, raise HDL as well.

11. Eat healthful oils from such sources as nuts (almonds, Brazil nuts, and walnuts), and olive and sesame oils. As we saw in the previous chapter, polyunsaturated and monounsaturated fats speed up the burning of adipose fat, enhance weight loss, create satiety, and boost immune function. They can also lower LDL and raise HDL levels.

Preventive tests

- Total cholesterol should be below 150 mg/dl, but as Dr. Topol points out, cardiologists now view total cholesterol as largely insignificant, since the LDL is the primary cholesterol culprit, and total cholesterol does not reveal exactly what the LDL number really is.

- Triglycerides, or blood fats, should be no higher than 150 mg/dl, and preferably much lower.

- Homocysteine. Normal levels range from 4–12 micromoles per liter of blood (expressed as umol/l), but cardiologists routinely request that it be 10 umol/l or lower.

- Fibrinogen. Normal levels range from 200–400 mg/dl, but most cardiologists like to see it well below 350 mg/dl.
- C-reactive protein. Another test that Dr. Topol and other authorities recommend is called C-reactive protein (CRP), which measures overall inflammation that may be occurring throughout the body. C-reactive protein is produced in the liver. When the liver is enflamed, due to the production of inflammatory compounds produced in the liver or elsewhere in the body, C-reactive protein levels rise. Like LDL and HDL, C-reactive protein can be measured with a simple blood test. Safe levels are 0.5 mg/dl or lower.

Heart disease is the greatest killer today, but ironically it is the most preventable illness we face. By implementing the most important lifestyle changes, including stopping smoking, maintaining a regular exercise program, optimizing nutrition, and addressing the underlying causes of the illness—inflammation and insulin resistance—we can not only significantly reduce our risk of heart disease, but we can also reduce our risk of diabetes, cancer, Alzheimer's, and so many other threats to our lives.

CHAPTER 7

The Biology of Cancer

The path to cancer

This year, more than 1.5 million Americans and more than 14 million people worldwide are expected to be diagnosed with cancer. We have all read a lot on the subject of cancer, heard from the experts, and searched online. We hope that this chapter sheds new light on the perplexing subject of cancer, which oftentimes escapes early diagnosis and presents without overt symptoms. According to the National Cancer Institute, obesity and inflammation are associated with many forms of cancers including breast, colon, pancreatic, kidney, endometrium, and others. They often occur silently, until the malignant cells override the body's immune and health-supporting systems. Studies have shown that insulin—and more specifically IGF (insulin growth factor)—plays a role in cancers and, more specifically, abetting their aggressiveness.

Takes many years

What we don't realize is that many of the changes that lead to cancer—especially the most common ones, such as breast, prostate, colon, lung, endometrial, and ovarian cancers, take many years to develop enough that we become aware of them. The initial process is often a genetic mutation that sets off a cascade of changes in our biology through some of the processes discussed in this book, such as inflammation or the use of hormones such as insulin. Increasingly, scientists are seeing the onset of cancer as a series of stages in a degenerative process.

Several cases of cancer are due to hormones and oncogenes—genes that transform healthy cells into cancer. Insulin is a known mitogen, meaning it triggers the reproduction of cells and the growth of tissues. Insulin and sugar play important roles. One thing we know for sure is that cancer cells love sugar, the cocaine of the masses. Researchers from Princeton University have found that with ingestion of large amounts of sugar, the brain undergoes changes similar to those seen in people who abuse illegal drugs like cocaine and heroin. "Our evidence from an animal model suggests that bingeing on sugar can act in the brain in ways very similar to drugs of abuse," says lead researcher and Princeton psychology professor Bart Hoebel.

The history of cancer

Going into 2017, we are witnessing the war on cancer at an inflection point of an arsenal with words such as "immunotherapy," "targeted therapy," and "CAR-T-cell therapy" (chimeric antigen receptor T-cell therapy), which are having profound effects in early data. But each scientist and doctor knows that this war possibly started 2,400 years ago, when the Greeks used the word Καρκίνος, or Karkínos, meaning "crab-like disease." From that Greek word we inherited the Latin derivative and the word became Cancer. Hippocrates and Galen and other nameless doctors of their time are some of the original warriors who tried expunging techniques and spiritual chants to remove the crablike growths. What is undoubtedly true is that each modern day scientist stands on the shoulders of those who preceded them. Take a moment and visit the American Cancer Society website and witness names like Giovanni Morgagni from the 1760s in northern Italy, or John Hunter from Scotland in the same century, Johannes Müller from Germany in the 1800s, or his student Rudolf Virchow, who coined the term "leukemia" in the early 1900s. Katsusaburō Yamagiwa and Kōichi Ichikawa from Japan tested cancers in animals, several decades later. The name that stands out is the remarkable Sidney Faber, considered to be the father of modern chemotherapy. Centuries of curiosity from diverse parts of the world laid the groundwork for major advances. The collective efforts of thousands of scientists from dozens of countries who all speak the same language of humanity and science will ultimately conquer this disease. Knowledge is power, and the more we talk about the advances in cancer treatment and the factors involved in the disease the better. There is a scene in Neil Simon's movie *Brighton Beach Memories* where the word "cancer" is whispered by the older generation, as if it were something to be ashamed of. Luckily today that is no longer the case.

Do lifestyle factors play a role?

As much as we know about genetic mutations and the pathophysiology and causes of illness, there is still a long way to go to a full understanding of why some people get cancer. Although it would be arrogant for doctors and scientists to think they have the answers, we do know the powerful role of lifestyle choices.

Although several of the biological links between cancer and lifestyle factors remain unknown, our understanding of how this disease comes about is advancing rapidly.

A sedentary state together with highly processed foods rich in calories and fat combine to create a set of harmful disorders: insulin resistance, weight gain, metabolic syndrome, and chronic, low-grade inflammation, all discussed in previous chapters. These disorders themselves release a horde of poisonous substances that change the way cells behave and function. These factors are often the underlying conditions that alter cellular and genetic behavior and may form the basis for cancer. Many of our daily behaviors create these conditions. However, once these disorders are in place, they set off a series of events—a kind of domino effect—that gradually poisons the body and destroys our defenses.

Eventually, they can alter gene functions and even possibly form the basis for malignancy.

We can control the amount of exercise we do and cut back on time spent on digital devices and watching TV. Studies from Nielsen and the Kaiser Family Foundation demonstrate that teens are watching 20–40 hours of TV a week. How many reruns of *How I Met Your Mother, Friends, The Voice, The Bachelor*, etc. can a person watch? And studies from the CDC and the Division of Preventive Medicine at Brigham and Women's Hospital reveal that less than a quarter of these adolescents get even one hour a day of physical activity. This inactivity leads not only to an increase in all the metabolic conditions and possibly type 2 diabetes, but also to it all occurring at a much earlier age.

In China there are 114 million people living with diabetes, a soaring increase from 1% of the population 25 years ago to approximately 11.6% of the population. This pattern is similar in India and Japan; due to an increase in Western-style diets but also physical inactivity.

Why cancer remains undetected!

A full-blown cancer takes years—and in some cases more than a decade—to develop before it can be detected by medical instruments or physical examination. That means that a very serious disease has gone unnoticed by the immune system.

"The genius of cancer is that it hides in the body while it grows, and then it becomes increasingly difficult to treat once it can be detected," said Edmundo Muniz, MD, PhD, a former vice president of Eli Lilly Research Laboratories Global Oncology Program, and current CEO and president of Certara. He is widely regarded as one of the world's leading experts on cancer and its treatment.

"In the early growth stages, cancer looks to the immune system like something created by the body, and therefore part of a natural process," he said. "This means that the immune system does not attack the cancer, because it does not recognize it as a threat. But once the cancer becomes strong enough, it overwhelms the immune system and then it is very difficult to treat."

In this way, cancer bears some similarities to HIV (human immunodeficiency virus), the basis for AIDS. "HIV learned from cancer," Dr. Muniz said. "Viruses use the genome from cells to grow. HIV looks to the immune system like other cells. Cancer is similar in this regard. Cancer cells look to the immune system like normal cells that are in revolution. From an evolutionary point of view, revolution has often been seen as a good thing. It's a kind of advancement of our ability to survive, and therefore seen by the body, including the immune system, as a forward movement. But cancer cells do not perform any life-supporting activity. They consume the life of the body."

Failure to commit cell death

Once the body wakes up to the presence of cancer, it starts signaling the malignant cells to die. It does this by initiating a process of programmed cell death called apoptosis. Unfortunately, the abundance of these free radicals in the system has brought about mutations (genetic changes) in the cancer cells, essentially allowing them to act independently from the overall system. One of the most important of these mutations is the degradation of a key gene known as p53, often referred to as the guardian of the genome.

What is P53?

P53 watches over cellular behavior and, when needed, tells cells to enter a phase of cellular repair. If cells cannot repair themselves, p53 orders the cell to initiate programmed cell death, or apoptosis. One of the first things cancer does is turn off p53. That means that when neighboring cells order the cancer to either repair itself or initiate programmed cell death, it can disobey.

In addition, cancer develops certain armoring characteristics that, over time, make it more resistant to chemotherapy. In effect, it learns how to adapt to the hostile conditions of the chemotherapy, making it even more difficult to treat. This is why recurrence of cancer—that is, cancer's return after it has been forced into remission by chemotherapy—is so difficult to treat. It is actually a far more virulent disease the second time around.

As you know, if allowed to proliferate, cancer cells are virtually immortal, or, at the very least, will live as long as the host patient survives. Scientists are searching for ways to "reboot" p53. A UCLA researcher may have stumbled upon a way to do just that.

The sugar toxin

It is now fully accepted that cigarette smoking is a clear cause of lung cancer, but excess sugar intake may also be toxic to our cells. And yet we consume pounds and pounds of this white poison.

According to a 2011 report, researchers from the CDC and Emory University studied thousands of teens' sugar consumption rates over the course of five years. They discovered that the average teen consumes 28 teaspoons of added sugar per day. The American Heart Association recommendation is a maximum of 5–8 teaspoons. Sugar and highly processed foods have an addictive effect on all of us. We have accepted this as "the normal way to eat." Yet the cells of our body struggle with these foods, which we have only been eating for the past 60 years and are unlike anything we have eaten in human experience before. The daily behaviors of inactivity and poor nutrition that we do without thinking inevitably lead to inflammation, insulin resistance, and—if allowed to progress far enough—metabolic syndrome.

Degeneration goes on and on

Tens of millions in America and hundreds of millions worldwide have allowed the degeneration to go on for too long. As discussed in the previous chapters, one in four adult Americans have metabolic syndrome, which is characterized by overweight (especially around the middle), high insulin, high blood glucose, high LDL cholesterol, high triglycerides, high blood pressure, inflammation, and low HDL cholesterol. It's easy to see why this disorder is so threatening to your health: the body is flooded with poisons—high cholesterol, insulin, glucose, triglycerides—as well as suffering from high blood pressure. These toxins and disorders, in turn, lead to high levels of inflammation, which releases an overabundance of free radicals in the blood and tissues. Free radicals, or oxidants, are highly reactive oxygen molecules that in most cases simply kill cells, but in some instances deform them. Very often, those deformed cells combine to form scar tissue, or nonfunctioning tissue that can appear anywhere in the body. Cataracts are but one example of the scarring caused by oxidants in the bloodstream.

However, in a high-oxidant environment, hordes of free radicals bombard DNA, killing many cells and causing mutations in others. Some of those mutations can trigger the onset of cancer.

Why is excess body weight a problem?

And then there is the added burden of too much body weight, which is created, in part, by high insulin levels due to overeating. When blood sugar becomes too high, the body converts those sugars into blood fats, or triglycerides. Insulin then forces those triglycerides into fat cells, thus making us fatter.

Adipose tissue—ordinary body fat—is highly active, producing an array of cytokines. When we are overweight, that fatty tissue produces many destructive cytokines, including tumor necrosis factor and IL-6.

"Fat cells are very active," said Pinchas Cohen, MD, the Dean of the Davis School of Gerontology University of Southern California. "There's lots of products going out of them, and most of them are bad."

Excess estrogen as a trigger

One of the more dangerous byproducts of fat cells is the hormone estrogen, which at high levels can be extremely toxic. In normal levels and in balance with other hormones, estrogen is a magnificent hormone that keeps all female bodily functions in great condition.

But at high levels, estrogen can act like growth hormone, causing tissue to grow rapidly in the hormone-sensitive organs, such as the breasts, uterus, ovaries, and prostate. These growing tissues can block blood and lymph vessels in these organs, causing blood and waste products to accumulate and stagnate. At the same time, rising estrogen levels can also be highly inflammatory. (During ovulation, when estrogen is surging, women often suffer from swollen, inflamed, and painful breasts.) Sometimes these inflammatory conditions go overboard and alter DNA, and may even trigger the onset of cancer.

These are some of the reasons why overweight and obese people have many times the risk of cancer than those who maintain a normal, healthy weight.

In a study published in the *Journal of Obesity* in August 2013, authors Giovanni De Pergola and Franco Silvestris reported that overweight and obesity dramatically increases the risk of chronic illness, particularly the most common cancers. Another study, published in the *Journal of the National Cancer Institute* in December 2008, by Kerlikowske, Walker et al., reported that overweight and obese women may have up to twice the risk of contracting breast cancer than women who are at their ideal weight or lower.

Unfortunately, overweight triggers cancer in other ways, as well.

Expanding fat cells produce a lot of "bad" products, as Dr. Cohen so aptly put it. On the other hand, lean adipose tissue does something extremely important—it creates *adiponectin,* a substance that actually fights cancer.

The hero hormone

Adiponectin is one of the heroes inside our bodies. Among the many things it does is block blood vessels from connecting to tumors. Thus, it deprives tumors of blood and oxygen, which is essential for their survival. This talent, referred to by scientist as *anti-angiogenesis*, is considered one of the Rosetta Stones of cancer research. Scientists are searching feverishly for ways to trigger anti-angiogenesis, which, in essence, would give them the ability to isolate tumors and cut off their blood supply, thus causing them to die.

Remarkably, adiponectin also triggers apoptosis in cancer cells. Animal studies, including one published in *Pharmacological Therapeutics* in May 2013, reported that not only did adiponectin remarkably prevent new blood vessel growth to tumors, but it also triggered a "cascade activation" that led to cancer cell death, and "significantly inhibits primary tumor growth." Finally, adiponectin significantly increases insulin sensitivity in cells, which means it helps take the body out of insulin resistance.

Clearly, a higher level of adiponectin in the bloodstream is desirable. And the way to get it is, very simply, weight loss. As weight goes up, adiponectin levels go down, thus increasing our vulnerability to all the diseases and disorders it protects us from. On the other hand, when weight drops, adiponectin levels rise, thus providing protection from cancers and other diseases caused by cells multiplying unchecked.

One such study, done by Dr. James Hebert and his colleagues at the University of Massachusetts (UMASS) Medical School showed that women with breast cancer who are overweight, or who gain weight after diagnosis, experience a much shorter life expectancy than those who keep insulin low and lose weight.

Hebert and his coworkers found that just eating an additional 100 calories per day over the standard 1,200-calorie diet increased the risk of recurrence by 5%.

Low adiponectin levels may be especially dangerous to women for another reason—they are associated with a particularly powerful form of cancer. Numerous studies have been published by Japanese researchers Miyoshi et al., including one published in the *Journal of Breast Cancer Research and Treatment* in December 2008. That study reports that "tumors arising in women with the low serum adiponectin levels are more likely to show biologically aggressive phenotypes. The association between obesity and breast cancer risk might be partly explained by adiponectin."

Adiponectin has been found to play a role in a wide array of cancers, including that of the colon, rectum, prostate, and endometrium.

The good news is that adiponectin levels can be restored rapidly, usually within weeks of adopting a diet and lifestyle that causes weight loss.

Insulin and growth hormones—a toxic cocktail

The human body is an awesome symphony of chemical and cellular functions, each one dependent on many others to remain in balance and in health. At the center of that symphony is insulin.

Insulin is itself a mitogen, or a substance that stimulates cells to replicate. Scientists have shown that when elevated, insulin can act as a trigger and actually fuel cancer proliferation. A good example is the BCL2 gene, now recognized as one of the genetic causes of several types of cancers, including breast cancer. Not all women who have the BCL2 gene get cancer. But those who have the gene, and maintain high insulin levels, are at much greater risk. Why?

When high blood levels of insulin are sustained over time, cells can develop a specialized BCL2 receptor on the cell membrane. And in an insulin-resistant environment, BCL2 receptors proliferate. That receptor, which acts as an antenna for the swarming insulin in the blood, is linked directly to the BCL2 gene inside the cell's DNA. Once insulin catalyzes, or phosphorylates, the receptor, it lights up a kinase cascade that turns on the BCL2 gene, which in turn initiates the cancer.

Women who maintain normal or healthy insulin levels are less likely to have the BCL2 receptor.

When elevated, insulin causes the liver to produce more growth hormone, including a specific type known as insulin-like growth hormone, or IGF-1. In youth, growth hormones, including IGF-1, become elevated in order to promote physical development and create normal-sized adults. But as we age, we don't need as much growth hormone any more and, consequently, the body reduces its production of IGF-1 and other growth factors. This is important because growth hormone causes cells to multiply and for tissue to get larger—which is exactly what a quiet small cancer needs in order to become a full-blown malignancy. Growth factors trigger cell division and multiplication—in essence, they promote cancer. One of the ways the body keeps growth hormone low is by keeping insulin levels in check.

Keeping insulin in check was something our ancestors didn't need to think about. Nature protected our forebears by limiting their menu and demanding lots of physical activity. No matter where humans lived, they all ate diets that were relatively low in fat and rich in plant foods. (Consider that even the animals that our ancestors ate were lean—approximately 4% body fat, according to researchers S. Boyd Eaton, MD and Kenneth Konner, PhD, whose 1985 study on Paleolithic nutrition was published in the *New England Journal of Medicine*. Compare that to the modern hamburger, which may derive up to 50% of its calories from fat. The USDA suggests that the maximum fat content for a burger should be 30%

Our ancestral diet was rich in unprocessed plant foods and low in calories, which meant that it kept insulin levels low. At the same time, our ancestors were forced to maintain active lives—especially because many early humans lived as hunter-gatherers, and later as farmers. Physical activity burns calories and keeps insulin levels low. As insulin levels fell in adulthood, so too did growth hormone levels and overall weight. Few, if any, of our ancestors had to think about dieting and aerobic exercise.

But modern life has created exactly the opposite conditions. Calories are high and physical activity is low. This causes insulin levels to rise, which in turn stimulates the liver to produce higher levels of growth hormone, especially IGF-1.

An ever-increasing body of evidence is showing that as insulin and IGF-1 go up, so too do the rates of breast, prostate, and colon cancers. "IGF-1 is one of the keys to cancer, especially cancers of the breast, prostate, and colon," said Dr. Cohen. "IGF-1 is a stimulator for cancer. There is associated data that show that as insulin levels go up, as IGF-1 goes up, so too does inflammation. These conditions also promote the generation of proinflammatory cytokines, which in turn promote numerous diseases, including cancer."

Making cells behave differently

James Barnard, PhD, a professor of physiological science

at UCLA, has been studying the relationship between diet and health for more than 30 years. Tall and athletically built, Barnard was, for much of his adult life, a long-distance runner, but in recent years he has slowed down to a daily, hour-long walk in the Southern California hills.

Among the populations of people Dr. Barnard has studied are those who come to the Pritikin Longevity Center, a center for the treatment of heart and vascular illnesses in Santa Monica, California, and Ventura, Florida. More than 90,000 people have been treated at the medically supervised Longevity Center, mostly for heart disease, diabetes, high blood pressure, claudication, and gout. The Center's primary form of treatment is the use of a diet that is composed of low-fat animal foods, whole, unprocessed grains, vegetables, beans, and fruit. In addition, the daily exercise program is made up largely of walking, yoga, and other gentle forms of exertion.

Dr. Barnard, who has published more than 200 peer-reviewed papers, has been examining the before-and-after effects of the Pritikin diet and exercise program on these people. Among the many studies Barnard has done on the Pritikin participants is the effects of a low-fat, low-calorie diet and exercise on insulin, IGF-1, and prostate cancer.

In Barnard's published articles, including one in the *US Journal of Urology* in 2010, he and colleagues found that men with prostate cancer who adopted an essentially low-fat, plant-based diet experienced a dramatic drop in insulin levels and insulin-like growth factor (which has same damaging effects as insulin when too high). The men also experienced an increase in the two important proteins that bind with insulin-like growth factor and take it safely out of the body.

These findings might have been anticipated, but what Barnard also found was not. Doing blood assays, Barnard found that, soon after adopting the diet and exercise program, the cancer cells in the prostate went into programmed cell death, or apoptosis. Essentially, the cancer started to die.

Scientists have been searching for decades for ways to trigger apoptosis in cancer. They have long known that one of the problems with getting cancer to perform apoptosis was the degradation of p53 gene, and they have been researching how could it be revived. Barnard believes he found one of the ways to do that.

"The drop in insulin levels caused the liver to produce less IGF-1," Dr. Barnard said. "At the same time, the diet and exercise program also raised the clearing proteins causing a further drop in IGF-1. These factors created the conditions for the initiating of apoptosis in the cancer cells."

The effect of diet and exercise on triggering cell death

In further studies, Barnard found that a diet low in fat and rich in unprocessed plant foods alone brought about a drop in insulin and IGF-1, and triggered apoptosis. Interestingly, exercise alone also triggered an increase in apoptosis. When combined, diet and exercise had an even more powerful therapeutic effect, causing even greater levels of apoptosis.

Many recent studies have corroborated these findings.

Increasingly, scientists are finding that appropriate diet and exercise lowers insulin, IGF-1, and brings about apoptosis in cancer cells. This new understanding may be among the reasons why Asian men with a diet low in saturated fat and sugar and high in fish and beans have much lower rates of prostate cancer than American men do. Moreover, when Asian men suffer prostate cancer, the disease does not become a malignant, but remains asymptomatic and confined to the prostate gland. Many Asians with prostate cancer die in old age, never knowing that they had the disease.

Some scientists believe that, similar to prostate cancer and IGF-1, breast cancer may sometimes be triggered by these tumor-promoting growth factors. Women with chronically high insulin and IGF-1 may have higher rates of breast cancer than women who have lower insulin and normal IGF-1.

New medical approaches to treating cancer

Not surprisingly, the advances in our understanding of cancer have led to new approaches in its treatment. Although some treatment regimes may elicit a complete remission, most chemotherapy approaches have been viewed less as a cure and more as a means of gaining time. This is hopefully changing slowly. One of the shortcomings of chemotherapy, doctors recognize, is that it actually weakens the body's own efforts to fight the disease.

"Chemotherapy can slow the growth of cancer by killing cancer cells," said Dr. Muniz. "But chemotherapy kills both cancer cells and immune cells. In this way, chemotherapy is like antibiotics, which kill both bacteria and healthy cells. But one of the reasons antibiotics work is because they are not strong enough to kill the immune system. The immune system is still intact and can assist with the work of antibiotics to kill the bacteria."

With chemotherapy, both the cancer and the immune system are weakened, but the cancer is able to rebound more rapidly, in part because the chemotherapy itself creates the conditions for the cancer's rebirth.

Once administered, chemotherapy leaves in its wake enormous quantities of free radicals, which can trigger additional mutations in DNA and bring about the rebirth of the disease. Free radicals also fire the embers of any surviving nests of old cancer, thus bringing them back to life.

"In the Middle Ages, people were hit by a two-by-four over the head as anesthesia so that they could extract a tooth or be operated on," said Dr. Muniz. "That's basically what we're doing with chemotherapy. Chemotherapy kills everything—the cancer and also healthy cells. In essence, we're hitting people with two-by-fours. The person is half dead and half alive from the treatment itself. And unlike with antibiotics, we cannot count on the immune system to help us fight the disease. Thankfully, [we know so much more about cancer today] and we're moving beyond that kind of treatment."

The future will bring entirely new approaches, Dr. Muniz says. Today we know so much more about the genetic makeup of cancer, and the person who suffers from the disease, that we can tailor a specific treatment for a person's unique genetic makeup.

Dr. Muniz says that new drugs are now being designed

to directly interfere with specific kinase pathways within the cancer cell, and in the process destroy the disease. One of those pathways is known as the EGF, or epidermal growth factor pathway. Dr. Muniz points to two drugs, Iressa and Tarceva, now being used effectively to treat cancer. "These drugs attach to the EGF pathway and stop cell division," Dr. Muniz said. "We are finding that they are working extremely well in people with lung cancer."

Another such drug now being used successfully Gleevec, which blocks the enzyme that fuels the growth of chronic myelogenous leukemia (CML). Before Gleevec, the average survival rate for people with CML was 4–6 years. On Gleevec, only 16% of patients with CML have relapsed, and many physicians believe that the drug will stretch the lifespan of people with CML up to 20 years.

Gleevec is also being used to treat people with gastrointestinal stomach cancer, which happens to be driven by the same enzyme as CML. Prior to Gleevec, there was no effective treatment for gastrointestinal cancer, with the average patient surviving only 1–2 years after diagnosis. More than half the patients treated with Gleevec are currently showing no signs of disease.

The targeting of specific kinases also opens up the possibility that scientists may be able to insert specific commands to cancer cells. One of the commands scientists are most eager to give cancer cells is the order to commit suicide.

What is immunotherapy?

New approaches in immunotherapy and targeted therapy

are showing great promise in blood cancers like leukemia and lymphoma, and hopefully eventually in solid tumors. This therapy uses the body's immune system to fight cancer cells and leave normal healthy cells alone. New terminology, such as "checkpoint inhibitors," is mentioned at every cancer conference. These inhibitors are like radar jamming that intercepts and disrupts signals between cells.

Immunotherapies fall into three general categories: *checkpoint inhibitors,* which disrupt signals that allow cancer cells to hide from an immune attack; *cytokines,* protein molecules that help regulate and direct the immune system; and *cancer vaccines,* which are used to both treat and prevent cancer by targeting the immune system.

Can food be therapy?

Scientists have learned a great deal about how foods affects us on the cellular and even genetic levels. Many superfoods, such as resveratrol in grapes, are being extensively investigated. One of the most promising of those foods is green tea. At the Medical College of Georgia, cell biologist Stephen Hsu, PhD, has been studying green tea for more than a decade. He and others have found that the antioxidant in green tea, epigallocatechin-3-gallate, or EGCG, triggers the flow of protein messengers that force cancer cells to differentiate. If they are unable to do so, the antioxidant instead initiates programmed cell death.

Michael Wargovich, PhD, a longtime cancer researcher at the South Carolina Cancer Center in Columbia, SC, points out that, "In tumors, certain signal pathways become corrupted and stop functioning so that the cells keep growing. It's like having the light switch taped in the 'on' position. When that happens in cells, certain functions become degraded and, in time, deplete the machinery and can cause some cells to become cancerous. Green tea reregulates the cell; it reboots the system, so to speak, to accept the command to stop growing."

At the very least, green tea is worth drinking for its anti-inflammatory powers. Because most diseases today involve inflammation, green tea may provide some protection against heart disease, diabetes, arthritis, and Alzheimer's disease.

Other foods affect genes in ways that also protect us from cancer. Soybeans and soybean products are a good example. Soybeans, scientists have found, stimulate the activity of 123 genes in the prostate that combine to suppress inflammation, tumor growth, and initiate DNA repair. Curcumin, a substance found in the spice turmeric, inhibits genes from triggering inflammation, which forms the basis for breast, colon, and prostate cancer, as well as Alzheimer's disease. The people of India are the highest consumers of turmeric per capita; they also have the lowest rates of Alzheimer's disease in the world.

At UCLA, David Heber, MD, director of the UCLA Center for Human Nutrition and a professor of medicine and public health at the UCLA Medical School, urges people to eat more plant foods as a way to add antioxidants and to combat inflammation. "A number of colorful fruits and vegetables have natural dietary agents that are antioxidant and anti-inflammatory," he told us in an interview. "The most evidence exists for soy protein, turmeric (containing curcumin), resveratrol (found in red wine), pomegranate ellagitannins, tea polyphenols from green tea and black tea, aged garlic extract, and lycopene from tomato products." Dr. Heber recommends that people eat a diet of five to nine servings per day of fruits and vegetables in order to get adequate quantities of antioxidants and other plant chemicals that reduce inflammation.

The power of the mind

Dr. Heber also points to our mental state as a powerful factor in healing. He recalls the experience of famed financier and former junk bond maven Michael Milken, who was diagnosed with terminal prostate cancer in 1993 and is not only still alive, but (and despite the scandal) thriving and healthy.

"The most powerful immune organ in the human body is the brain and central nervous system," said Dr. Heber. "I believe that an individual can influence disease processes. I have seen too many people die within a year of the death of a spouse or within a year of retirement to discount the impact of mental function on health. We are a long way from proof, but I believe that there is an individual healing process not reflected in our large cancer studies that predict mortality. With a PSA of 24 and a Gleason score of 9 [both indicating the presence of virulent cancer], Michael Milken statistically has outlived every prediction and beaten prostate cancer. Was it his diet, his medical treatment, his mental determination or a combination of all three?" Dr. Heber believes it was a combination of all three plus more.

CHAPTER 8

Why Stress?

Universal disorder

Everyone has stress. It is indeed the universal disorder. Life equals stress. We feel overextended and overwhelmed, constantly trying to attain the elusive work-life balance as we juggle all our commitments. You can no more eliminate stress from your life than you can eliminate tension from your muscles. If muscle tension dropped to zero, you would fall to the ground in a shapeless heap. If all stress disappeared, you would not function. It's only when it becomes overwhelming that it becomes problematic. You need some "good" stress in order to thrive. Unfortunately most of your life circumstances push you into overwhelming, simmering stress. And it's this negative stress that causes all the harm.

The sources of stress in our lives seem endless, but

most of them are related in one way or another to time, or the lack of it, and all too often we're late. Caught in traffic or behind on some deadline, and pushing ourselves to our limits. We're all in a rush to get someplace. Been on the West Side Highway in NY after a Yankees game, or the Grand Central Parkway during a Mets game, perhaps the FDR to JFK during rush hour, or the Santa Monica Freeway I-10? It doesn't matter where in the world you find yourself—the streets of Delhi, Bali, and Honolulu all suffer from traffic jams. Caught in traffic, behind on some deadline, and pushing ourselves to our limits, we feel that simmering stress.

Every moment, it seems, is filled, spoken for, or scheduled. And every new technological advance—e-mail is just one example—seems to steal more time and make new demands. In the twenty-first century, progress all too often means more stress.

Stress takes its toll

It's taking a toll. The World Health Organization predicts that by the year 2020, stress-related disorders will be the second leading cause of death in the world. The physical and mental disorders arising from stress on the job now costs US businesses more than $300 billion annually in productivity and health care costs.

Stress, especially when it's chronic, is dangerous for two reasons. First, it can cause profound and often destructive changes in our biochemistry. It may weaken the immune system, damage the heart, and even alter neurons responsible for memory.

One of the most important ways that stress affects our health is by elevating insulin levels, and keeping them elevated, eventually resulting in weight gain, insulin resistance, and all those conditions that flow from metabolic syndrome, including diabetes.

Second, it often causes us to engage in coping behaviors that are themselves dangerous to our health. People under stress are more likely to smoke cigarettes, drink alcohol to excess, and eat foods high in fat and calories. For many people, the methods used to cope with stress are as destructive as the stress itself.

Stress has become a major source of illness today. To combat stress we need to understand how it affects the body and determine what we can do about it.

The threat!

Implicit in every stressful situation is the recognition that something valuable is threatened. And therein lies one of the keys to understanding stress. When it comes to assessing a threat, stressful situations are in the eye of the beholder.

Sonia Lupien, PhD, is one of the world's leading experts on stress. As the director of the Center for Studies of Human Stress at McGill University's Douglas Hospital Research Center in Montreal, Canada, she has studied the effects of stress on people of all age groups, from the very young to the very old.

Dr. Lupien is French-Canadian and speaks English

with a distinct French accent. She presents much of her information as historical analogies and human stories, rather than the dry facts of science.

Absolute vs. Relative Stress

"We live in very secure countries, relatively speaking," said Dr. Lupien. "We're not living in Iraq or Darfur. Yet, according to the World Health Organization, most of us are going to be dying from stress-related problems. How is this possible? The answer is that the human body cannot tell the difference between real stress (an absolute stressor) and apparent stress (a relative stressor)."

An absolute stressor, according to Dr. Lupien, is a situation in which our lives are clearly in danger. Relative stressors, on the other hand, are those that threaten our status, identities, or livelihoods. Unfortunately, the human body cannot tell the difference between the two, which means we often experience the same physiological reaction to the experience of being stuck in traffic and late for a meeting with the boss as we do when we face a life-and-death situation.

Part of the reason for this is simple: throughout most of our existence, humans have faced absolute stressors, meaning situations in which our lives really were in grave danger. Our bodies adapted to these fears by developing biological mechanisms that would give us the best chance of surviving.

"In prehistoric times," said Dr. Lupien, "we had to kill the mammoth in order to feed the tribe. So we were forced to come face to face with the mammoth, and that was surely an absolute stressor. You could be killed facing such a beast. Your body wants to survive. Part of you wants to run away from the beast, and another part wants to eat. Your brain knows this, it sees the danger, and therefore signals a stress response."

The biological response

The biology of that response is now well understood. At the recognition of danger, the hypothalamus, an endocrine organ located in the brain, releases a substance called corticotrophin-releasing hormone (CRH). The CRH triggers another gland, the pituitary, also located in the brain, to secrete a second hormone called adrenocorticotropin (ACTH).

ACTH travels in the bloodstream to the adrenal glands, located above your kidneys, and signals them to release *adrenaline* as a first line of stress and then a group of stress hormones. The first of these are known as *glucocorticoids* (the most widely known of which is *cortisol*); the second are known as *catecholamines* (specifically epinephrine and norepinephrine). These substances combine to increase heart rate, respiration, and smooth muscle function. Blood is diverted away from central organs and into muscles, getting us ready for intense physical action. At the same time, blood sugars and fats that are stored in the body are released into the bloodstream so that they can be utilized for energy. In the face of rising glucose and blood fats, insulin levels spike to open up cells to the abundance of fuel that's suddenly available.

This highly potent cocktail of hormones, blood fats, glucose, and insulin triggers the well-known "fight or flight" response, which is part of our survival instinct. Suddenly you can run faster, jump higher, lift heavy objects, and fight for your life.

"The beauty of the system is that when you faced the mammoth, or some other threat to your life, your body responded by giving you the energy you needed to fight or flee," said Dr. Lupien.

"Because the human body does not make a distinction between an absolute stressor, or a relative stressor," Dr. Lupien continued, "all the same biochemical events that happen when we face the mammoth also happen when you are sitting in your car late for a meeting." Except one, and it's an important one.

"The difference is that when you face a mammoth, you are going to need a lot of energy, and you're going to expend a lot of energy," she points out. That means that all that glucose, and all those triglycerides that are released into the bloodstream in the face of a threat are now going be burned as fuel. The fight or the flight is going to utilize all the glucose that your body has suddenly made available to you. When the fight or flight is over, you're going to be hungry for food, because you just expended all your energy reserves.

"But when you're sitting at your desk and receive an e-mail that the deal has fallen through or in your car and experiencing stress at being late, your entire body gets ready for the intense stress response with muscles and heart poised for action. In addition, that glucose and fat that are suddenly available in your bloodstream are not going to be burned as fuel," said Dr. Lupien. "Instead, they're going to cause your insulin levels to rise. You may burn a little, but the rest you're going to store as fat." This is the first step in a process in which stress actually increases our weight.

For the person experiencing stress while sitting in his car, the increased levels of glucose and blood fats are also going to drive up cholesterol levels, which are going to have an adverse effect on the heart and arteries. You may have adapted to such chronically high levels of stress that you now assume this state to be normal.

Stress as a cause of weight gain?

As if all of this were not enough, another survival mechanism kicks into gear, much to the modern person's detriment. His brain believes that he just faced the mammoth, or the saber-toothed tiger, and consequently has expended all his energy. That means that the brain is going to cause him to think he's hungry, which means he's going to eat more, even though he's got an overabundance of fuel that he'll have to store in his tissues as fat.

"The same hormones that combine to give you energy, the glucocorticoids, have this strange property of going back to the brain and telling the brain that you've just expended energy and you need to eat," Dr. Lupien said. "The glucocorticoids are steroids and capable of crossing the blood-brain barrier within minutes of experiencing stress. Once the stressor has passed, they signal the brain that energy has been burned and must be replaced."

This is one of the reasons why people eat so much when

they are under chronic stress, which is the case for so many of us today. Our bodies believe that we have been foraging for food, or facing down some hostile creature that had to be killed in order for us to survive.

We also eat to relieve the tension that is stored in our muscles as a consequence of the stressor. A study done by Tanja C. Adam and Elissa S. Epel, published in the medical journal *Physiology and Behavior* (April 2007) reported that "a subgroup, possibly around 30%, decreases food intake and loses weight during or after stress, while most individuals increase their food intake during stress." Adam and Epel report that most people not only increase food intake, but choose foods that are especially dense in calories. For most Westerners, that means choosing processed foods such as pastries, bagels, chips, or bread, or choosing foods that are rich in fat, such as ice cream, chocolate, cheese, and other dairy products. "The combination of high cortisol, dense calories, and consequently high insulin contributes to the visceral fat distribution," Adam and Epel report. By visceral fat, they mean the fat that's around your waist.

In the belly!

We needed calories when we faced the mammoth, but we also needed them in a place where they could be rapidly mobilized and made available to us in seconds. Evolution found just the place for those fatty calories—your belly.

"The body doesn't know about our ideas of beauty or health," Dr. Lupien says. "On the contrary, it says, 'Listen, you have a lot of mammoths in your life—that's why you're always in the stress response. You need a lot of energy to fight them off, which means you're going to have to eat a lot and store as many calories as you can."

Whenever you are under chronic stress, your brain will create regular bouts of hunger, even when your body has plenty of stored energy. And it will store those excess calories on your belly as a form of rapidly available, emergency energy.

The consequence of these two survival mechanisms—increased hunger and accumulation of calories around your waist—is overweight and potentially obesity.

As Dr. Lupien puts it, "The body says 'I figured out that if I store the glucose and fat in my abdomen, then I can use it faster.' This is why we, in the field of stress research, see abdominal obesity as a good marker for chronic stress. Other factors change, as well. Heart rate is definitely going to increase. So, too, does cholesterol."

The sudden availability of blood fats is going to drive up cholesterol levels. But there's another reason cholesterol goes up. The body needs cholesterol to make hormones, including stress hormones, which means that the more stress the body experiences, the more it will need cholesterol in order to make stress hormones. "So if your body needs a lot of stress hormone, you will need to eat foods that increase your cholesterol levels," said Dr. Lupien.

As weight, triglycerides, cholesterol, and insulin levels rise, so too does inflammation. Now you have the foundation for a whole host of illnesses, including diabetes, heart disease, many forms of cancer, and other serious illnesses. (See previous chapters on metabolic syndrome, heart disease, etc.)

"There are many studies that show that an increase in glucocorticoids will lead to an increase in insulin, and insulin resistance, which will then lead to an increase in type 2 diabetes," Dr. Lupien said.

Going "NUTS"!

One of the problems we face in the twenty-first century is clearly identifying what constitutes an actual threat—in other words, a truly stressful situation—versus a situation that only appears to be threatening, but really isn't. In short, we haven't figured out yet when to be stressed out, and when to relax. Some of this is due to our biology, and some of it is our failure to adapt.

Hans Selye, the pioneer Canadian stress researcher, first identified the stress response in 1936. Selye spent most of his time researching physical reactions to stress, such as the effects of heat and cold on the body and nervous system. Based on his research, Selye extrapolated that any stressful situation could cause a stress response.

But in 1968, psychologist John Mason came along and questioned Selye's theory. He said that the body can adapt to stress, especially when a stressful situation is repeated over time. Mason did a series of experiments in which he monitored the stress hormones released by people under a wide variety of stressful situations. Among his subjects were a group of people who parachuted out of airplanes. Mason studied both the men and women who jumped for the first time, as well as instructors who had made such jumps dozens of times.

Mason found that, right before they went into the airplane, the first-time-jumpers experienced acute escalations in stress hormones. Mason thus concluded that jumping from airplanes is, indeed, highly stressful. But then he found something interesting. The trainers stress levels remained normal when the got into the plane and even made their jumps. For them, jumping out of an airplane was routine. Not only was it routine, but it didn't represent a significant threat to the trainers. In other words, there was no reason to be afraid, as far as they were concerned.

"The first time jumpers didn't know what to expect," said Dr. Lupien. "For them, this was a frightening experience. Moreover, they didn't feel in control of the situation. The trainers, on the other hand, did know what to expect. They didn't feel it was especially dangerous, and they were in control." From these experiments, Mason came up with a set of four criteria that formed the foundation for a stressful event. All four characteristics do not have to be met, Dr. Lupien said, but the more of them that are met, the more stressful the situation is.

Those four characteristics are as follows:

1. Novelty. The situation must be new to the person, and therefore foreign. The less we know how to behave in situations, the more stressful they are.
2. Unpredictability. The outcome of the event must be unpredictable. When something is at risk and we are uncertain as to how the situation will unfold, the more stressful it is.
3. Threat. Something we value must be at risk to

KASH, FRIEDLAND, & LOMBARD

be stressful. When a situation poses a threat to our lives, our livelihoods, or our identity, it is considered stressful. It's important to remember that identity can include our status and our ego identification with the outcome of a project or situation. The person who is known for always being on time can experience a great deal of stress if he is stuck in traffic.

4. Sense of no control. Situations that pose a risk and are out of our control are inherently stressful. And the greater the risk, and the more out of control the situation seems, they more stressful they are.

Using the first letter in each of the four criteria, Mason coined the term NUTS as the basis for interpreting whether or not a situation was stressful.

As Dr. Lupien points out, we face situations every day that we interpret as a threat to our identities or our livelihoods, which means most of us are dealing with NUTS on a daily basis.

That is especially the case at work, where stressful situations seem to arise on a daily basis. According to the American Institute of Stress, 80% of American workers say that they feel stressed on their jobs, and nearly half say that they need help coping with stress. 62% of workers say that they routinely end the work day with work-related neck pain, and 34% say that stress disrupts their ability to sleep at night.

Stress, Insulin, And Cancer

Leroy Morgan, MD, PhD, is the retired head of the pharmacology department at Louisiana State University in New Orleans. He has also worked closely with the National Institutes of Health to develop an array of pharmaceutical agents to treat disease, including drugs to treat cancer. In addition to being a long-time researcher at LSU, Dr. Morgan is a general practitioner, seeing patients for more than 30 years and has observed much about health and disease which don't arise from textbooks. He has observed first hand the relationship of stress and cancer. Because as stress raises insulin levels, it also causes a sharp increase in insulin-like growth factor, or IGF-1, which in turn promotes the life of malignant cells and tumors.

"When a person experiences negative stress, the body causes a breakdown in fat and carbohydrate stores, which causes glucose levels to spike and insulin levels to go up," Dr. Morgan says. "Prolonged stress leads to chronically high insulin and IGF-1 levels, which in turn may make a person vulnerable to cancer."

Dr. Morgan also takes into account the fact that when people are under stress, their diets and exercise habits tend to change. Very often, more fat, processed foods, and alcohol are consumed, all of which increase insulin and IGF-1 levels.

"I have seen that a major stressful event, such as divorce, bankruptcy, job loss, or the sickness or loss of a loved one, may cause a dramatic change in blood chemistry," Dr. Morgan said. "Then 18 months to two years later, a person may even be diagnosed with cancer."

This does not mean that all major life stressors lead to cancer. It certainly does not mean that if you have cancer, it was a big life stress that set it off. It is simply another piece in the huge puzzle of factors that may contribute to cancer.

Coping with Stress

If stress elevates important blood constituents, and may contribute to the conditions that give rise to major illness, the best way to combat stress is to burn fuel and to burn the adrenaline simmering away in the body. We must, in effect, turn off the adrenaline so that the body can shift into a relaxation phase where healing and repair can take place.

Exercise is the single most important factor in switching off adrenaline after using it up. Once we begin exercising, the first reserves of fat that we will burn will be in our muscles, our livers, and in our stomachs. Stomach fat is quickly mobilized and made available to our cells whenever our energy levels fall, especially when we are using our muscles in any from of exertion. The body is going to surrender that stored energy very rapidly during exercise.

"Whenever I am under stress, I run," Dr. Lupien said. "The reason is simple. I know my body is going to start storing calories as fat, and that's going to have a big impact on my health. So I have to increase my exercise to burn off the calories that my body is going to accumulate. In effect, I have to do something physical that would burn calories as if I were fighting the mammoth. So whenever my neighbors see me running, they know I'm under stress."

A half hour of vigorous exercise per day is all it takes

to burn the fat that has accumulated on the body, and particularly around the middle. Perhaps the best program for exercise is to combine some form of vigorous exercise, which you do a few times a week, with a more gentle form, such as a half hour a day of walking. If you do not have a half hour per day, do three ten minute walks. The research shows that three ten minute walks have an accumulating effect that amounts to that 30 minute walk.

The best way to get some form of vigorous exercise is to find a game or a practice that you really enjoy. Consider taking up tennis, racquetball, or volleyball, or perform a martial art, or do aerobic or ballroom dancing, swing, or tango, or run on a treadmill—and do it at least three times per week. The FIT principle is a good way to remember—*f* for frequency; at least three times a week, *i* for intensity; at a moderate level and *t* for time for at least 35–40 minutes. Yoga is typically thought of as gentle exercise, but anyone who does yoga regularly knows it's a workout. Try doing some yoga three to five times a week, and couple it with a daily walk. You'll find your condition will begin to improve rapidly.

In addition to that walk or enjoyable, vigorous practice, be active every day. Walk up the steps to your office, or take short walks from your car to your office. Get your heart rate up, even for a few minutes, to improve circulation, engage your muscles, and move your body.

Exercise alone can lower insulin levels, build muscle, and burn fat. And in the process, it can protect you from the range of serious illnesses that arise from high stress and high insulin.

On the other hand, serious consequences result if

changes in behavior—especially exercise and diet—do not occur in the face of chronic stress. Dr. Lupien points out that chronic stress, along with chronic elevations in insulin, can lead to various kinds of adaptation, including chronic adaptation to stress with very high levels of cortisol or what scientists refer to as dysregulation in the brain. Dysregulation of brain function that is sustained over time can lead to neurological dysfunction.

Metabolic syndrome, stress, and depression link

In the human body, nothing happens independently. Everything is connected to everything else. The human mind cannot fathom the awesome orchestration of trillions of cells, each performing multiple tasks, and all of them woven together into a moving tapestry that is both orderly and creative at the same time. As you've no doubt noticed, that tapestry gets scrambled by metabolic syndrome.

Among the relationships that scientists have recognized consistently is that people with metabolic syndrome often suffer from heart disease as well as depression. As researchers looked more closely for clues as to why insulin resistance might be associated with depression, they found an interesting fact turned up again and again. People with metabolic syndrome have low serotonin levels.

Serotonin is responsible for creating within us a sense of well-being and confidence. When elevated, serotonin gives us the ability to concentrate, to focus on a given subject, and to relax and enjoy deep sleep. When serotonin is low, we can experience increased anxiety and, if it falls low enough, even depression.

Most of the antidepressant drugs are referred to as "selective serotonin reuptake inhibitors," or SSRIs. These drugs work by increasing brain levels of serotonin, and thereby lower depression.

Serotonin can also be elevated by exercise, a consistent healthy sleep routine, and meditation and mindfulness. If, after implementing these techniques into your life, you still feel really low, reach out to your doctor and get some help. Oftentimes even with the best intentions and best strategies you will still require SSRI antidepressant medication for a period of time to alleviate the depression. They work extremely well and are not at all habit forming.

The Golden Years?

We are generally living longer compared to any other time in history. Some data demonstrates that the elderly are more satisfied than the younger generations and certainly not as intensely stressed. They are no longer bound by the same time urgencies. However, the 70-plus generation experiences a different type of life stress than the young and robust. Many feel very lonely and isolated. Several studies show that even though only about 28% of seniors over the age of 65 live alone, over 40%, acknowledge that they feel lonely. The number one stressor for elderly is the disintegrating family unit. Unfortunately in many cases, there is loss of contact. In a study by Iowa State University, 10% of mothers are estranged from a child later in life, meaning no communication. The good news is that with internet calls and low-cost phone calls more people speak regularly to their isolated parents. A 2013 study by AARP (American Association of Retired Persons) showed that today more than 30% of baby boomer children call their senior parents every day compared to a generation ago, when that number was only 13%.

Stress from the death of a spouse is high but so is caring for the long term health issues of a partner, especially Alzheimer's and dementia. An interesting finding in the study of caregivers (those looking after an ill spouse) is a significant rise in a biomarker of inflammation and illness called interleukin-6 (IL-6). This means that the body is in an inflamed state, which can cause potentially significant damage to cells. Some studies have shown up to a four-fold increase of IL-6. This also affects other biochemical and structural changes affecting longevity, lifespan, and memory.

A unique study involving more than 800 priests, nuns, and brothers known as the Religious Orders Study at Rush University's Alzheimer Center showed that stress produces higher levels of cortisol, which effects memory, and that the more emotional distress the higher the rates of Alzheimer's disease.

In today's economy, financial stress is a major pressure affecting mental and physical well-being.

Teenagers and stress

Throughout the world, teenagers are constantly attached

to their digital devices, updating Facebook, Snapchat, Instagram, Twitter, Viber, WhatsApp, and of course Tinder, all the while under pressure from school, college, work, and peers! Whatever happened to time spent outdoors and knowing it was time to get home for supper by looking at the sunset?

They face piles and piles of homework, huge expectations from parents and teachers to perform, a fast-changing world and an epidemic of teenage depression and anxiety. What often escapes us is that teenagers' lives can be just as stressful as our own. One of the major challenges for teens today, in the US and globally, is the scourge of bullying. According to the US Department of Health and Human Services almost a third of all students experience some type of bullying in school and 70% witness bullying, 43% of students ages 11–17 have false rumors spread about them on social media, 36% experience some form of pushing, and 32% experience being hit or kicked. The saddest stat is that 160,000 students miss school each day for fear of being bullied.

But this phenomenon is not just reserved to the United States or the West. A 2016 study of 5,000 students by the China Youth and Children Research. Center collected some eye-opening data: 33% of students surveyed experienced some form of bullying and 6% experienced severe bullying. In Europe, Austria has the highest rate of bullying according to a 2010 study by the Organization for Economic Cooperation and Development at 20%, and Sweden the lowest, at 4%.

Go to bed!

Add to this scenario the fact that teens just do not sleep well. Maybe on a quiet remote island a youngster is getting a good night's sleep. But for the rest, they are seriously sleep deprived. Diana Paksarian et al. in the *American Journal of Public Health* (July 2015) demonstrated that only 40% of 15-year-olds got at least seven hours of sleep—almost 60% had even less. This is a worldwide problem. Japan seems worst, with an average of only six hours of sleep. A recent Pew Research Center study showed that 72% of teenagers bring their cell phone into their bed and most leave it on all night.

Explosive brain growth, rewiring, and neural reorganization

Adolescence is not just a period of dramatic physical growth and sexual development but moreover a time of explosive brain development. Much of their behavioral changes are due to significant reorganization and "rewiring" of the brain structures.

Science in the form of brain imaging has changed our understanding of adolescence.

Until fairly recently, we had no idea just how profound the brain changes are during adolescence. Research in the past decade has revealed that the brain undergoes significant reorganization and suggests that teens aren't intentionally making bad choices or being careless or stressed out.

Dramatic brain reconfiguration takes place in an area called the prefrontal cortex. This is the reasoning part of the brain, responsible for clear thinking and decision making, and it undergoes a process often referred to as pruning. Areas of this critical brain structure are being rewired, making the brain more efficient. Some connections (called synapses) are literally whittled away or sloughed off, making way for new and stronger connections. The prefrontal cortex is also wired into the limbic system, the emotional part of brain that helps us make sense of the world and relate to others. The thinking processes are often thrown off course by activity triggered in the emotional part of the brain. A simple explanation for adolescent moodiness is that the thinking part of the brain has not yet developed to the point where it can rein in the intense reactions of the emotional brain. Dr. Laura Kastner, a clinical professor of psychiatry and behavioral sciences at the University of Washington, explains in her book *Getting to Calm: Cool Headed Strategies for Parenting Teens and Tweens* (2009) how neuroscientists characterize the risks inherent in teen years as a big engine, poor driving skills, faulty brakes, and high-octane fuel. The big engine refers to the brash new push for autonomy, poor driving skills result from the reconstruction of the teens' prefrontal cortexes, faulty brakes describe the teens' lack of impulse control, and high-octane gas refers to the intense emotions accompanying adolescents' hormonal changes.

Why stress—kids just lose it!

It is bewildering for parents to observe the extreme mood fluctuations in their teenager. But rest assured that, for the most part, mood swings are quite typical of adolescence. They are an unavoidable side effect of the dramatic physical, hormonal, and brain transformations taking place. Recent groundbreaking research demonstrates that teenagers' petulant behavior and mood swings are due to unexpected chemical reactions in their developing brain. Scientists have found that the mechanism normally used by the brain to calm itself down in stressful situations seems to work the opposite way in teenagers, explains Dr. Sheryl Smith of the State University of New York in *Nature; Neuroscience* (March 2007). The effect of these changes is that whatever the teenage person's reaction to stress is likely to be, whether it is to cry or be angry, the reaction will be amplified. "While to adults it may seem like an overreaction, to the teenager it is the only thing they can do," says Dr. Smith.

This study is thought to be the first to suggest an underlying physiological—as opposed to a behavioral-psychological—explanation for teenage mood swings. You may well be concerned as to whether the mood swings are more serious than other adolescent changes. But unless your teen's angry, depressed, or anxious mood continues over an extended period of time, there is no reason to be overly concerned. Whilst parents tend to overreact, Dr. Smith suggests the following: Don't interrogate your teen by firing off questions like "What's wrong with you?" They don't know what's wrong. Instead, acknowledge that you can see they are having a hard time and make yourself available to talk. If they don't want to talk, back off and allow home to be a safe, comfortable, and nonjudgmental environment. Suggest some of the simple yet smart techniques that we should be using such as breathing techniques, going for a run or brisk walk when overwhelmed, going outdoors and getting some fresh air, the use of calming music, and best of all, learning to meditate.

Is it just a mood swing or real depression?

Most teenagers experience depressed moods at times. It is completely normal and common during adolescence, more so than at other life stages, to feel depressed intermittently. Your teen may feel low or even depressed about lots of things: love relationships turned sour, difficulties at school, troubles with friends. They feel awful when life just seems to get tough; they feel overwhelmed and stressed. Sometimes there is no apparent reason. If the depressed mood occurs occasionally and most of the time she feels generally good, there is usually not much to worry about. However there is cause for concern if she is in a depressed state most of the time. There are signs other than the low mood to watch out for. If she shows a loss of interest in friends and fun activities and becomes angry and irritable, if her grades start slipping and she generally withdraws, these might be indicators of depression. If she loses her appetite or overeats, has insomnia or sleeps all the time, it is time to seek professional help. Many of these signs might also indicate regular use of marijuana.

If you suspect that your teen is depressed, it is a good idea to approach a mental health professional or your GP. If your teen talks about just wanting to die, take it seriously and seek help immediately. Dr. Garry Walter, chair of the Child and Adolescent Psychiatry Department at the

University of Sydney, believes that there are various ways that parents can assist their depressed teenager. Walter suggests that "a parent can keep the GP or counselor informed about the child's progress, encourage the child to persevere with treatment, try to minimize levels of stress in the family, and be openly hopeful—after all, in the vast majority of cases, the outcome is very good." He suggests that we take depression seriously. Offer unconditional love and concern. Let the teen know you are present and available for them without being pushy. Support them and encourage them to get help.

Take action if it is a frequent or constant problem and seek out the help of a professional. It is probably best to discuss the problem with your family doctor first. Teens mostly tend to keep things to themselves but you should be at hand and receptive to listening if they do want to talk. If your teen won't go for help and you are worried, go yourself first and get advice on how to best handle the situation.

Take seriously any talk about suicide.

CHAPTER 9

Alzheimer's, Memory Loss, and Dementia

The darkness of Alzheimer's disease

Few aspects of aging are more terrifying than the specter of having your mind swallowed whole by the darkness that is Alzheimer's disease. Anyone who has witnessed a loved one's slow withdrawal into that lost and unreachable realm knows. Alzheimer's is a mind robber. Gradually, inexorably, it steals your memory and your sense of self until all of those whom you have loved, and all who have loved you, become part of a parade of passing strangers. Past, present, and future are a blur. The memories and relationships that define you as a unique person collapse and disappear in the dim mists of dementia.

Alzheimer's disease is a neurological disorder that causes

the slow, progressive loss of memory. It is also accompanied by confusion, withdrawal from social contact, gradual loss of speech, emotional agitation, uncontrolled muscle movement, incontinence, and often hallucinations. People with Alzheimer's are losing brain cells—in effect, their brains are shrinking—and with such losses go memory and other cerebral functions.

The illness can last as long as 25 years, but usually causes death within 8–10 years of onset. It was originally diagnosed by German physician Alois Alzheimer, who recognized two abnormal characteristics in the brains of people who were afflicted with the disease: the presence of amyloid plaques—essentially scar tissue in the brain—and the twisting of microtubules, also known as *neurofibrillary tangles,* which, in health, allow nutrients to flow within nerve cells or neurons. When these tiny tubules become damaged, or twisted, the flow of nutrients ceases and the cells die. Great swaths of gray matter are lost in the Alzheimer's-afflicted brain, along with the brain's ability to produce adequate quantities of a chemical neurotransmitter known as acetylcholine, which is essential to experiencing memory.

Standard Dementia vs. Alzheimer's

These symptoms, which characterize Alzheimer's disease, contrast with the more common form of dementia, which usually arises when the brain is deprived of oxygen. In common dementia, atherosclerosis has caused the diminution of blood flow to crucial areas of the brain, causing brain dysfunction and memory loss. Standard dementia is not associated with the extensive swaths of amyloid plaques and neurofibrillary tangles that are seen in patients with Alzheimer's disease.

The numbers are rising dramatically!

Alzheimer's disease currently afflicts some 4.5 million Americans, or 1 in 10 over the age of 65. Nearly half of all Americans 85 and older have Alzheimer's.

The number of people with Alzheimer's disease is now exploding. In the 1980s alone, incidence of Alzheimer's rose 1,000%. Physicians are quick to point out that part of that increase is due to heightened awareness—doctors are more likely to label dementia as Alzheimer's today. Nevertheless, leading researchers in the field point out that even when increased awareness is taken into account, the numbers of people showing up with Alzheimer's is rising dramatically. Health experts predict that by the year 2050, more than 14 million Americans will suffer from Alzheimer's. Like so many other rising illnesses—metabolic syndrome and diabetes, for example—this one poses a tremendous threat to our health care system.

One of the many aspects of Alzheimer's that make it so frightening is that researchers do not understand how it develops. While different theories abound, many scientists would say that the cause of Alzheimer's is essentially unknown. Complicating the picture is the fact that genetic research has revealed that only 15–20% of all Alzheimer's cases are considered purely genetic in origin—that is, the consequence of inherited traits passed down from parents and ancestors. But new and persuasive clues have been mounting, and due to the work of leading scientists a clear picture of the causes of Alzheimer's has started to emerge.

Insulin's role in the brain

Over the past few years, it has become clear that insulin plays a role in brain function. In addition to regulating appetite, it is now appreciated that insulin signaling is crucial for learning, memory, behavior, and survival of brain cells. Insulin activates critical brain neurotransmitters, including dopamine and acetylcholine. Insulin resistance is linked to diminished levels of dopamine and acetylcholine, possibly leading to addiction, obesity, ADHD, and Alzheimer's disease.

Alzheimer's disease: a form of diabetes?

Alzheimer's, many scientists now believe, may even constitute a form of diabetes of the brain. Indeed, one of the world's leading Alzheimer's researchers, Suzanne de La Monte, MD, PhD, of Brown University Medical School, is now referring to Alzheimer's disease as type 3 diabetes— meaning a type of diabetes that destroys brain cells and leads to dementia.

"In Alzheimer's disease, brain cells cannot respond to insulin appropriately," Dr. De La Monte told us in an interview. "Neurons, like all other cells, require insulin to produce ATP (the fuel used by cells). If they cannot respond to insulin, normal energy production, metabolism, and cell signaling doesn't happen, and among the things you get is low production of acetylcholine."

This revelation has opened doors to new and possibly effective therapeutic avenues. Researchers have found that inhaled insulin may improve memory in normal, elderly people. Inhaled insulin is now being considered as a potential treatment for Alzheimer's disease.

Not only are these revelations leading to new forms of treatment, but scientists are recognizing new approaches to prevention. Clearly, prevention measures begin by recognizing the need to keep insulin levels under control, and by avoiding metabolic syndrome and diabetes.

People with diabetes are twice as likely to develop Alzheimer's as nondiabetics. The same amyloid plaques that build up in the brains of Alzheimer's victims appear in the pancreases of diabetics. Moreover, researchers say when metabolic syndrome is added to the picture—that is, overweight, high blood pressure, high glucose, and high insulin levels—the risk of Alzheimer's skyrockets.

A study done by Rachel A. Whitmer and her colleagues at Kaiser Permanente in Oakland, California, followed more than 22,000 patients for eight years. The participants who developed full blown diabetes had the highest risk of Alzheimer's. In fact, those with the highest blood sugar levels had an 83% greater risk of contracting Alzheimer's than those whose blood sugar levels remained normal.

Insulin levels are directly related to weight. As insulin rises, so too does weight gain. It's for this reason that the overwhelming majority of people with type 2 diabetics are overweight. Following this strong connection, Dr. Whitmer did another study in which she followed 10,276 men and women for seven years. As she and her colleagues found, those people who gained the most weight in middle age had the greatest risk of developing Alzheimer's disease. Of those who became overweight in middle age, 35% developed Alzheimer's later in life. Of those who became obese, 74% developed Alzheimer's.

Not only are overweight and obesity indicators of rising insulin levels, but they are also associated with high blood pressure and high cholesterol—in short, metabolic syndrome, which researchers have found dramatically raises the risk of contracting Alzheimer's disease. One study found that people who are overweight and borderline diabetics—in essence, those who suffer from metabolic syndrome—were 70% more likely to get Alzheimer's than lean nondiabetics.

There are 41 million Americans with metabolic syndrome, all of whom are possibly at increased risk of contracting Alzheimer's. Not all of them will get Alzheimer's, of course—in large part because many will die from some other insulin-related illness, such as heart disease, cancer, or a stroke, or from other complications stemming from diabetes.

Turning Neurons into Scar Tissue

Dr. De La Monte has been exploring the link between brain levels of insulin and Alzheimer's disease for much of the past decade. A neuropathologist and associate professor of pathology and medicine at Brown Medical School, Dr. De La Monte is one of the pioneers in revealing the link between insulin resistance and Alzheimer's. Indeed, her research won her the prestigious Alzheimer's Award in 2000 for making the year's outstanding contribution to our understanding of the disease.

Beta-Amyloid

Among the questions that have baffled researchers are: Why do the brains of those who suffer from this illness accumulate a toxic protein, known as *beta amyloid*? All human brains produce this protein, but people with Alzheimer's disease do not clear the protein from the brain. Instead, it accumulates and eventually forms amyloid plaques, which disrupt neuron signaling and eventually cut off production of acetylcholine.

Another question is: Why do the neurons in Alzheimer's patients become twisted, or tangled up, into these convoluted masses of inert tissue?

In her search for answers, Dr. De La Monte and her colleagues examined the brains of 45 deceased people who suffered from Alzheimer's disease and compared them to the post-mortem brains of people who had not suffered from the illness. What the researchers found was startling. The Alzheimer's-afflicted brains showed significantly fewer insulin receptors on their neurons, indicating that insulin could not be taken effectively into cells. Without insulin, cells die, but not before undergoing dramatic and destructive changes.

"Those with the most advanced Alzheimer's disease had nearly 80% fewer insulin receptors than normal brains," said Dr. De La Monte. The researchers also discovered that as insulin levels in the neurons fell, neurons died and Alzheimer's disease progressed.

Insulin growth factor (IGF-1)

Insulin wasn't the only essential substance that was lowered inside of neurons. So too was insulin-like growth factor, or IGF-1. Contrary to what goes on in cancer, where too much IGF-1 can stimulate tumor growth, the human brain requires IGF-1 in order to support neuron function. Not only does IGF-1 stimulate cell growth, but in the brain it makes neuronal connections more complex, thus allowing for more complex forms of thought to take place. Growth factors are part of the reason human brains are capable of learning and thinking creatively.

However, without adequate numbers of insulin receptors on the neurons, brain cells cannot absorb adequate quantities of insulin and glucose. Nor can they be stimulated by IGF-1. Declines in insulin, glucose, and growth factors cause gradual reduction in neuron function and eventually cell death. People with Alzheimer's are losing brain cells—in effect, their brains are shrinking—and with such losses go memory and other cerebral functions.

Scientists are trying to understand why this brain loss occurs. In fact, although insulin isn't stimulating cells so that they absorb glucose, it is present in the brain, at least in the early stages of Alzheimer's disease. The insulin is not being absorbed by cells as it would in a normally functioning brain, in fact, in people with Alzheimer's, insulin is accumulating in the blood and tissue of the brain. Because high levels of insulin is toxic, the brain recognizes the excess insulin as a threat and utilizes a particular protein, called insulin-degrading protein (IDE), to clear the insulin from the blood supply.

The problem is that IDE is also used to clear beta-amyloid—the protein that leads to the creation of amyloid plaques which is turn disrupts brain function. In effect, the excess insulin competes with beta-amyloid for IDE. Unfortunately, the insulin wins—meaning it robs the brain of the IDE it would otherwise use to clear beta-amyloid.

That means that the more insulin in the blood, the less IDE there is for the brain to clear the beta-amyloid protein. As beta-amyloid accumulates, it creates plaques and scarring of brain tissue, which leads to the loss of acetylcholine, loss of memory, and cell death.

Neuron tangles

The accumulation of beta-amyloid is not the only destructive process that leads to Alzheimer's. There is also the creation of those twists and tangles that destroy the microtubule canals within neurons. Again, insulin resistance may set off a domino effect of damage of enzymes called kinases within cells that eventually lead to the tangling of neurons.

In a healthy brain, stable insulin levels raise a kinase within the cell called AKT. AKT in turn inhibits another kinase, found downstream from AKT, called GSK3. In effect, AKT is a good cop to GSK3, which can get out of hand if not restrained. Unfortunately, in insulin resistance,

AKT levels drop and GSK3 rises. In effect, the police force is weakened and the GSK3 gang gets stronger and goes wild. The elevated GSK3 levels overstimulate a protein known as tau, which is when damage to cells begin to happen.

Tau

Tau is the engineer of the microtubules inside your neurons. It helps grow and maintain these canals in which nutrients flow. But when GSK3 levels rise, they overstimulate tau, which cause the protein to misbehave. It's as if tau is over-stimulated, making it hyperactive and chaotic. The result is that tau turns those beautiful and orderly tubules into a tangle of weaves and meshes that destroy neurons, which die and cause the loss of brain function.

Ideally, GSK3 should be under the control of AKT, which keeps the kinase relatively quiescent. In that state, GSK3 gently supports tau. But in insulin resistance, both kinases become disrupted and all that orderly plumbing in the brain is turned into a jumble of disorganization that is reflected in brain dysfunction.

Stated simply, insulin signaling plays an essential role in the survival of brain cells. In insulin-resistant brains, the brain forms amyloid and tau proteins, the two destructive substances that form the basis for Alzheimer's disease.

Inflammation

The two best-known signs of Alzheimer's, in the brains of its victims, are the beta-amyloid plaques and the tangles of tau protein. But the disease also features chronic inflammation. Cells known as microglia which are the brain's cousins of the bloodstream's macrophages—swarm around amyloid plaques and dying, tangled neurons. They seem helpful, gobbling up beta-amyloid as well as disease-damaged cells. But their immunological enthusiasm also harms healthy cells, accelerating the disease. They may even be the initiating factor! Scientists have debated these questions for more than two decades. Now a burst of new research suggests that inflammation does, indeed, play a major role in Alzheimer's—and that targeting specific elements of that inflammation could be useful in treating or preventing the disease.

Inflammation: friend or foe?

Wherever it occurs in the body, chronic inflammation is a double-edged sword. The initial inflammatory response is meant to protect tissues against viruses, bacteria, cancer cells, and in Alzheimer's disease—from the harmful amyloid protein aggregates. But the longer it lasts, the more this inflammation stresses and kills healthy cells. Over time—as in rheumatoid arthritis, for example—the inflammation can become self-sustaining.

Extensive research has demonstrated that the chronic inflammation found in Alzheimer's hastens the disease process, and may even be a disease trigger.

Dr. De La Monte says that inflammation is occurring at the early stages of Alzheimer's, but researchers still don't fully understand all the sources of that inflammation. "Some kind of proinflammatory response is occurring as a consequence of the presence of macrophages and cytokines," Dr. De La Monte said, "but we don't fully understand the cause of the inflammation. The inflammation that's taking place in the brain is extremely subtle. If I hadn't measured it, I would not have seen it. But inflammation plays a critical role." Indeed, inflammation is part of the constellation of factors in the brain that are killing brain cells.

Possible triggers

High insulin is just one of numerous possible causes resulting in high levels of beta-amyloid. As it accumulates, beta-amyloid begins to decay, or break down, and in the process releases free radicals. These highly reactive oxygen molecules, in turn, cause the breakdown of cells, eventually destroying many neurons. Your immune system recognizes the problem and sends in macrophages to repair the damage. But in trying to restore health, the immune cells release cytokines—including interleukin-6—which are highly inflammatory. These chemical messengers call forth armies of additional immune cells, which release more free radicals and more cytokines. As crowds of immune cells gather, more inflammation occurs in the area, cutting off oxygen flow to cells and deforming and destroying more neurons.

The fact that inflammation is occurring at the early stages of the illness gives scientists some hope for an effective treatment. "Inflammation is occurring in diabetes, as with many other degenerative diseases," Dr. De La Monte said. "If you suppress it in diabetes, you may ameliorate the disorder. In the brain, you have inflammatory responses going on and they are taking place early on, so that if we could detect and reduce the inflammation, we might be better able to control the illness."

Inflammation, Vascular Disease, and Dementia

By killing neurons, inflammation can dramatically reduce brain function and acetylcholine production. But it also can trigger nascent Alzheimer's, or accelerate the early stages of the disease by reducing the blood and oxygen flow to the brain.

This is a new understanding of Alzheimer's—that it is often accompanied, and made worse, by atherosclerosis, or vascular disease, in the vessels that bring blood and oxygen to the brain.

Inflammation causes atherosclerosis in the carotid arteries, located in the neck, which bring blood flow to the brain; it is also the basis for high blood pressure, which injures arteries, as well. High blood cholesterol and high blood pressure combine to trigger an immune reaction, or inflammation, in the tissues of arteries and lead to the creation of artery plaques. Once those plaques grow large enough, they can block blood and oxygen supply to the brain. The result is impaired brain function, neuronal cell death, and eventually dementia.

Inflammation clearly occurs in pathologically vulnerable regions of the Alzheimer's disease (AD) By better understanding AD inflammatory and immuno-regulatory processes, it may be possible to develop anti-inflammatory approaches that may not cure AD but will likely help slow the progression or delay the onset of this devastating disorder (Haruhiko Akiyama, Steven Barger, *Neurobiology Aging*, 2015).

Two types of dementia at the same time

"Vascular disease is a contributing factor in the creation of Alzheimer's," said Dr. De La Monte. "When you look at the brains of people with Alzheimer's disease, what you find is that about 40% of them have Alzheimer's disease and vascular disease. They really have two kinds of dementia going on at the same time—Alzheimer's disease and what is called vascular dementia."

For those who may be in danger of developing Alzheimer's, vascular disease only increases the danger. "If you have a low level of Alzheimer's and you have a bad vessel disease, it can bring on the illness, or make it worse," said Dr. De La Monte.

Numerous studies have corroborated Dr. De La Monte's statement. A five-year study published in the *Journal of the American Medical Association* (November 10, 2004) that followed 2,632 men and women, all in their 70s, and all with metabolic syndrome, found that those with the highest levels of inflammation had the highest rates of dementia.

In a study published in the medical journal, *Neurobiology of Aging* (December 2005), Claude Messier et al. concluded, "Our data suggests that excessive insulin invokes synchronous increases in levels of beta-amyloid plaques and inflammatory agents, effects that are exacerbated by age and obesity. This constellation of events may have deleterious effects on memory." Other studies have had similar findings.

These links between inflammation and disease explain why people with metabolic syndrome are so much at risk for Alzheimer's disease and other forms of dementia. They have all the markers for increased risk of Alzheimer's, including high insulin, overweight, high blood pressure, and high cholesterol—all of which combine to decrease blood and oxygen to the brain and trigger the onset of Alzheimer's disease.

There is a silver lining. By recognizing that insulin resistance, inflammation, and vascular disease all play a role in the onset of Alzheimer's, doctors are offered an array of new approaches to hopefully try to prevent and treat the illness.

New Hope for Alzheimer's?

There are currently five approved therapies or medications for Alzheimer's, all showing some moderate efficacy in possibly slowing the progression of the disease, although as of yet there is nothing that can reverse the condition once it has begun.

Lifestyle and disease prevention strategies

One of the first issues researchers are encouraging people to recognize is that insulin resistance and overweight must be avoided at all costs. "Obesity in middle age increases the risk of future dementia," Dr. Whitmer concluded. She told the *New York Times* (July 17, 2006), that people must control their blood sugar levels throughout life, but this becomes especially important as we approach old age.

"Tight control is important for the whole life span," Dr. Whitmer said. "The older you are, the more likely you are to get dementia." This means, of course, that diets rich in calories and saturated fat must be avoided. Processed and fatty foods drive up insulin levels and lead to weight gain, insulin resistance, and type 2 diabetes. They also lead to atherosclerosis and artery disease, thus increasing the odds of Alzheimer's.

Dr. Whitmer offered a stark warning if such advice isn't heeded. "With the whole diabetes epidemic we're seeing much more type 2, so are we going to see even more Alzheimer's than we thought we would see. If we continue in this direction, it's a little frightening."

Keeping insulin levels within healthy ranges is essential. A diet rich in unprocessed plant foods and low-fat animal foods, especially fish, not only will keep your insulin and weight down, but it will also protect your arteries, and thus keep blood and oxygen flowing to your brain.

Researchers have noted for many years that Japanese people living in Japan have far lower rates of Alzheimer's and dementia than Japanese who come to the US and adopt an American way of eating. Japanese living in Japan eat diets that are rich in grains, vegetables, and fish, while those living in America eat a diet that's far richer in calories and animal foods, and thus saturated fat. Other differences in disease patterns between Westerners and Asians—especially in breast, prostate, and colon cancers—are consistent with this same finding.

This same trend has been found in Africans versus African-Americans—and not coincidentally, the latter have far higher rates of Alzheimer's. Rates of Alzheimer's vary greatly around the world and there is a probable link to the predominant diet in each area.

Researchers analyzed Alzheimer rates and dietary patterns in 12 different countries and concluded that "diet, dietary fat, and to a lesser extent, total energy (caloric intake) were found to be significant risk factors for the development of AD..., while fish consumption" significantly reduced the risk. Morris MC, Tangney CC, Wang Y, et al. in *Alzheimer's & Dementia* (February 2015) demonstrated that diets rich in whole grains and vegetables may lower the risk of the disease.

In a study entitled "Mediterranean Diet and Cognitive Decline," published in the scientific journal *Public Health Nutrition* (October 2004), researchers found that the standard Mediterranean diet—rich in complex carbohydrates from grains and vegetables, monounsaturated fats from olive oil, and red wine—was associated with much lower rates of age-related cognitive decline (ARCD) and dementia. They found that consumption of olive oil appeared to be particularly protective. "It cannot be excluded that the positive effect of dietary habits on cognitive functioning among healthy elderly subjects could be due in part to the antioxidant compounds of olive oil," wrote the researchers. Antioxidants reduce the rate of oxidation and lower inflammation. Virtually all plant foods are rich in antioxidants, as are high-quality plant oils, such as olive oil.

In a 2015 study Tanghey and Wang advocate for the MIND diet. This is a new diet developed by these researchers with elements from the DASH (Dietary Approach to Stop Hypertension) and MED diet, and also includes foods thought to protect the brain. It includes olive oil, whole grains, green leafy vegetables, berries, fish, poultry, beans and nuts, and a daily glass of wine, but restricts red meat and meat products, fast or fried food, cheese, butter, pastries and sweets.

In addition to diet, the activity that is most protective of your arteries is exercise. Exercise alone will lower insulin levels, create greater insulin sensitivity in cells, lower blood pressure, and lower inflammation. It also raises HDL cholesterol, which protects the arteries throughout the body. Alzheimer's researcher Dr. Weili Xu points out that exercise and diet combined can reverse prediabetes and may even help prevent dementia.

That was the conclusion of a study examining 1,740 healthy adults, 65 years and older, and published in the *Annals of Internal Medicine* (January 2006). The researchers Eric B. Larson, Li Wang, et al. found that those people who exercised at least three times per week were far less likely to develop any form of dementia, including Alzheimer's disease, than those who exercised less frequently, or not at all.

More and more researchers are looking at lifestyle factors as the underlying contributor to development of Alzheimer's disease. Noting that only a small fraction of Alzheimer's arises purely from genetic reasons, scientists are looking increasingly at daily diet and exercise patterns as a major factor. As the researchers of the Mediterranean diet concluded, "the prevalence of AD [Alzheimer's disease] is more strongly influenced by diet and nutrition, environment, and/or lifestyle than by genetics."

Such a revelation cuts both ways. While it reveals potential future health risks, especially if we persist in following a diet and lifestyle that supports insulin resistance, overweight, and diabetes, it also offers ways to protect ourselves and our loved ones from the illness.

Treating insulin resistance and its related disorders is not the only approach we can take, however. There are other steps that may protect us as well.

Exercise your mind

Studies have shown that those who keep up and maintain active learning well into their senior years have much lower rates of Alzheimer's disease.

"There's a lot of ways to look at this phenomenon," said Richard S. Jope, PhD, professor of psychiatry and behavioral neurobiology at the Miller School of Medicine, University of Miami.

"When you get Alzheimer's disease, you lose a lot of neurons before you experience any cognitive deficit," he said. "So people who read a lot may be the ones who started out in life with more neurons—they have a big surplus—so that they can lose a lot of neurons before they experience any sort of impairment. That's one way of looking at it."

On other hand, living a more intellectually challenging and adventurous life may be inherently good for the brain.

"Another way of looking at things is to see the brain as a muscle," said Dr. Jope. "And like any muscle, the same rules apply. Use it or lose it." In fact, scientists have found that learning stimulates brain cells to produce more growth factors, such as IGF-1, which sustain neurons and with them our ability to learn, to think complex thoughts, and to retrieve memories.

Numerous studies have supported this perspective. Scientists have found that a supportive environment, with ample stimulation and regular demands for learning new skills, may protect the brain from premature cell death.

A study published in *Cell* by Yeuchs and Steller (2011) showed that animals placed in environments that were both supportive and stimulating experienced much lower rates of cell apoptosis (cell death) within the brain than animals that were made to live in isolation. The researchers concluded that "a complex, enriched environment has important effects on brain function, by providing resilience to...insults [to brain tissue] as well as stimulating new cell birth and preventing cell death."

Similar findings have been shown in human research, as well. Those who achieve higher levels of education, and go on learning new skills well into their later years, have far lower rates of Alzheimer's and other forms of dementia.

Clearly, humans need to be challenged and to grow in order to feel alive. Such basic needs, born of tens of thousands of years of experience, may well be woven into our DNA. Among the lessons of Alzheimer's may be that without external stimulation and a pressing need to learn and adapt, the human brain atrophies and eventually dies. Evidence of this fact has turned up throughout human history.

In their book, *A General Theory of Love* (Vintage

Books, 2000), authors Thomas Lewis, MD, Fari Amini, MD, and Richard Lannon, MD, point to the experience of Frederick II, Holy Roman Emperor and King of Sicily in the thirteenth century, who instructed a number of foster parents and nurses to avoid all forms of communication with their children. The king believed that if he kept the children isolated from all forms of speech, they would spontaneously begin speaking the innate language of humans, which the king assumed would be either Hebrew, Greek, Latin, Arabic, or Italian. Unfortunately, all the children died before they spoke a word. A Franciscan monk who observed the king's experiment later noted that the children needed communication of all sorts in order to develop normally and stay alive.

Life is expressed by our need to learn, to share our inner thoughts and feelings, to experience connection with others, and to constantly grow from our experiences. Clearly, such adventures in learning are among the fundamental needs that keep us healthy and alive. When it comes to Alzheimer's disease, there are many other factors must be taken into account, as well. Among them are a healthy way of eating, engaging in physical activity, and maintaining a healthy weight. No doubt researchers will soon discover other important protective behaviors. In the meantime, what we have learned to date gives us a clear direction, and may be enough to protect ourselves, and those we love, from the multiple scourges that torment the body and destroy the mind, before they snuff out our lives.

CHAPTER 10

Children at Risk

The top health concerns for kids

Childhood well-being is of paramount importance not only to parents but also to the whole community. Our priorities as parents and concerned adults is to ensure our children and those within our communities are as healthy and safe as possible. We have a responsibility to ensure that children grow and develop in as healthy a way as possible, that they are up to date with immunizations, and that we are aware of the common and not-so-common conditions that may befall a child.

Although most of the common health issues facing children (in countries such as the US, UK, and Australia) such as common infections and allergies pose no real threat, there are alarming threats to their long-term health, from the epidemic of childhood obesity and diabetes to the dramatically increasing incidence of mental health issues.

A comprehensive review of all childhood illnesses is way beyond the scope of this book and therefore only a number of pertinent and worrying issues will be addressed. In the 2015 NPCH (National Poll on Children's Health) based on an annual survey of the top 10 health concerns facing kids in the US, adults rated childhood obesity, bullying, and drug abuse as their top three concerns. The C. S. Mott Children's Hospital in Michigan publishes this national US-wide poll annually and this year's results are as revealing as they come. The 2016 survey cites mental health issues as the number one concern. Overall, 7 of the top 10 concerns reflect children's mental health, either specific mental health problems (depression, stress, and suicide) or issues that often have an underlying mental health component (bullying, drug abuse, school violence).

Acute childhood conditions

Colds are a normal part of life and it is absolutely normal for your child to experience numerous viral colds and viral infections in their early years. These include episodes of vomiting and diarrhea, too. These diseases spread quickly but also settle fairly quickly. Be on the watch, though, for serious complications like extremely high fevers and unusual, extensive rashes. In those cases, see your doctor. A good rule of thumb is that any symptom in kids that doesn't settle within two weeks should get checked out.

Chronic childhood conditions

Children may develop a chronic condition in their early life. Chronic allergies and asthma are fairly common and there are rarer disorders such as chronic juvenile arthritis and type 1 insulin-dependent diabetes. Many of these can be very well treated and some children may even grow out of conditions such as childhood asthma. In the field of healthcare, children are not miniadults. Although with adults and cancer, there is often a strong link with possible lifestyle habits such as smoking, excessive alcohol consumption, or decades of poor nutrition, this is not the case for children. Cancer in children is generally due to a spontaneous genetic mutation and in no way within our control.

The chronic childhood condition that is certainly within our control is the alarming epidemic of childhood obesity.

Childhood obesity

At present almost one in three children in the US, UK, and Australia are overweight or obese. And the numbers are skyrocketing. This is the first generation of children who may have a shorter lifespan than their parents! Overweight and obese children have a much higher chance of developing heart disease and diabetes. They also have more emotional problems relating to confidence and self esteem.

Childhood obesity is associated with serious health problems and the risk of premature illness and death later in life. It is definitely a good idea to talk about the problem, and get it assessed by your doctor in a most nonjudgmental way. Your doctor or clinic nurse can plot your child's weight and height and work out a BMI (body mass index). Children do grow in spurts, so it is best to monitor and keep track. It is best to change the eating and activity patterns of the whole family rather than singling out the one child. Be sensitive to your child's needs; ensure you are embarking on a lifestyle change together.

Childhood diabetes

Type 1 diabetes is *not* associated with obesity or a poor lifestyle. It is an autoimmune condition where the pancreatic cells are damaged and can no longer produce insulin. This was the only diabetes seen previously in children. However type 2 has now become much more common in children and is associated with all the metabolic and cardiac risk factors. Ensure you are doing all in your power to encourage regular activity, a super-healthy eating plan, and excellent glucose control to ensure your child does not go on to develop further illness and complications.

Childhood Cancer

Leukemia accounts for about 25% of all childhood cancer. Discovering your child has leukemia is a terrible shock. Fortunately the chances of long term remission and possibly even a cure are possible. Brain and nervous system tumors are the second commonest cancer in children, accounting for another 20%. It is a frightening and traumatic experience to have a child be diagnosed with a brain cancer. In

2017, there is so much more that can be done than ever before. It is essential to garner an enormous amount of support from the medical team, psychologists, and counselors. Also harness as much support from family members and extended family as possible. Most pediatric centers have an integrated and comprehensive team of caregivers, nurses, and specialists to assist you through this trying time.

Children and mental health: Three childhood mental health narratives

Adam, an 11-year-old in the fifth grade, has brown hair, freckles, and is 18 pounds overweight. His parents refer to him as "stocky," but his physique clearly foretells the future—unless dramatic changes occur, he will battle weight issues for the rest of his life. That may be the lesser of his problems. As he sits at his desk at school, Adam is intensely restless and has great difficulty giving his attention to his school work for longer than 30 seconds. He fidgets with his pencil, looks over at his neighbor to his right, looks back at his teacher, and then to his neighbor on his left. His feet bounce up and down on the floor. He reaches for a piece of paper in his notebook and starts drawing impulsively on the paper. His expression remains detached and impassive, even when he draws a large X over the picture he has made. He raises his hand and asks his teacher if he can go to the bathroom. Permission is denied. He seems unaffected by his teacher's response, as if her words were never spoken. Instead he continues to look around the room, apparently searching for something to engage his attention for longer than 20 seconds. Adam suffers from attention deficit hyperactive disorder (ADHD), and this is one of his better days.

Nancy, 13 years old, has recently been weepy, lost interest in her schoolwork and activities, and is often lethargic. She has a poor appetite, wants to just sleep much of the time, and is extremely anxious about performing well at school. These changes seem to have surfaced since the onset of puberty and a diagnosis of mild depression and anxiety has recently been suggested.

Jimmy is nine years old and acutely sensitive to voices and noise. He is intensely shy and lost in his own internal world. When left to his own devices, he is clearly hyperactive and obsessive. If an adult attempts to speak to him, he refuses to look at the person, and when he does, he stares into the person's mouth, as if it holds some kind of secret that has nothing to do with the person's words. When Jimmy speaks, he often repeats phrases over and over again, like a mantra. He seems relieved when his mother holds his hand or touches his body. Jimmy has autism, a brain disorder that is characterized by social withdrawal, inability to communicate feelings and complex thoughts, and intense sensitivity to sensory inputs. All of Jimmy's outward behaviors are a reflection of his brain's anatomy.

When scientists examine the brains of autistic children, they find that certain regions are overdeveloped. The normal sculpting of the brain, accomplished in part by apoptosis, has not occurred, causing abnormalities in brain structure and function. For many people with autism, higher reasoning is lost and the perception of threats is exaggerated.

These children all suffer from distinct and different disorders, but their conditions share an underlying set of factors that may play a role in their origins. Researchers do not have all the answers as of yet, and much is still shrouded in mystery. But little by little, clues to the origins of mental disorders, such as ADHD, depression, and autism, are emerging. As they do, a coherent picture is starting to take shape, one that involves a complex array of genetic and environmental factors. There are obviously many social triggers that may exacerbate mental disorders especially depression. Experiences such as bullying at school, poor self-esteem, and social pressures are often enough to set off a mild depressed state in children. But oftentimes none of these factors are present, and at the heart of this picture is a combination of metabolic and neurochemical imbalances. All the aspects of systems biology may play a role, including brain chemistry changes due to inflammation, and even insulin resistance.

Depression in kids and teens

Childhood depression is real. It is normal for kids to feel sad and moody intermittently but this is not depression. When a child's sadness is persistent and ongoing and interferes with school and life—i.e. his functioning is disrupted—it may indicate that he or she has depression.

According to the Anxiety and Depression Association of America 80% of college students experience daily stress, 13% diagnosed with depression or anxiety disorder and 9% considered suicide in the past year. Depression is rife in high school kids and even in elementary school aged children. Data from the 2015 National Institute of Mental

Health shows that 8.3% of high schoolers suffer depression that lasts one year, compared to 5.3% of the general population. Results also show that 5% of students nationwide suffer from major depression and 10–15% suffer from varying levels of depression, yet only 33% seek help.

Do not ignore depression; it is not a fleeting mood or condition that will go away without treatment. Take it seriously. As with adults, children and teens with depression do well with psychotherapy but almost always requires medication too. It is essential that your child is monitored by a childhood- or teenage-specialist psychiatrist, who will keep a close eye on the effects and efficacy of the medication.

Take depression seriously; let your teen know you are present and available. Support them and encourage them to get help. Offer unconditional love and support even if it just seems like normal stress. Take especially seriously any talk of suicide and get help immediately, even if you think it is just a cry for help.

ADHD and ADD

Attention deficit disorder (ADD) and attention deficit hyperactivity disorder (ADHD) refer to a group of features associated with attention difficulties. The most common features include restlessness, impulsiveness, and inattentiveness (and hyperactivity). For a diagnosis the child should demonstrate these features both at school and at home. Not everything that presents with attention problems or hyperactivity is due to ADD or ADHD, however. Sometimes a hearing problem, reading problem, sleep deprivation due to enlarged tonsils or adenoids, or a chronic illness such as epilepsy, obsessive-compulsive disorder, or Tourette's syndrome may be misdiagnosed as ADD. A medical diagnosis and full assessment is required by a child psychiatrist, neurologist, or pediatrician.

Currently in the US, some 11% of children and 4.4% of adults now have a diagnosis of ADHD. While that ADHD is more common in the US, research points to an increasing global prevalence of ADHD diagnoses (7–9% of children) as well as an increase in consumption of ADHD medication. The cause is still essentially unknown, although there is a genetic component, and premature birth may be a contributing factor, or family stresses. But in most cases it is unknown.

Drugs and ADD/ADHD

Since 1990, the sale of Ritalin and other drugs used to control the disorder have jumped five-fold. Increasingly, children are being placed on extremely powerful drugs that, in some cases, have significant side effects. The medications certainly have side effects and should be prescribed only after a thorough assessment by highly trained professionals. Interventions including play therapy and counseling are advised, as well as following some well-described guidelines such as establishing boundaries, good routines, and schedules. Be specific with instructions and be consistent, try to remove distracting elements during homework time, communicate one-to-one with good eye contact and work together as a team with the schoolteacher. However, even with the best strategies, mediation is often still warranted. About 40–50% of children outgrow the problem, but the rest carry it through into adulthood.

The role of nutrition in ADD/ADHD

For decades, parents of children with ADHD have noticed that their children's behavior improves dramatically when they avoid certain kinds of foods, including those that contain sugar, milk products, artificial colors, flavors, or preservatives. In the early 1970s Benjamin Feingold, MD, an allergist who practiced in California, introduced the Feingold Diet for children with ADHD. The diet restricted all foods that contained artificial colors, flavors, preservatives, and salicylates, aspirin-like substances that Dr. Feingold said could affect moods in sensitive children. Other foods and food substances were called into question as well, including milk products, corn, and wheat. Parents who adopted the Feingold Diet said they saw immediate improvements in their children's behavior. In fact, communities and support groups sprang up throughout the country that swore by the effectiveness of Feingold's diet. Soon, scientific studies began investigating the approach.

To date, there have been 23 studies examining the relationship between specific food items and attention deficit and hyperactive behavior. "Some of these studies demonstrated significant improvement in the behavior of children when their diets were changed, or deterioration in their behavior when they were given food dyes or other offending foods," Eugene Arnold, a professor emeritus of psychiatry at Ohio State University told the editors of *Nutrition Action Newsletter*, a publication of the Center for Science in the Public Interest, a Washington DC-based public advocacy group (CSPI).

Indeed, in an earlier review of the research, CSPI found that fully 17 of the 23 studies had reported a clear relationship between certain food substances and ADHD behaviors. Only 6 experiments had found no connection at all, CSPI reported.

"It makes a lot more sense to try modifying a child's diet before treating him or her with a stimulant drug," Dr. Marvin Boris, a New York pediatrician, told CSPI.

Nevertheless, the food industry has seized upon the small doubt cast by those six studies to convince the general public that no relationship between food and behavior has been shown. Many medical experts today denounce the belief that food might play a role in either the onset or the severity of ADHD. They point to studies in which no relationship has been found between the two.

Part of the problem has been that science could not explain how food components might affect brain function. Another issue is that researchers could not explain why some children might be sensitive to these substances, while others do not react to them.

All of that is now changing, especially as scientists are able to understand how food and exercise affect glucose, insulin, and brain function.

Many researchers now believe that the relationship between food and ADHD may not be a straight line. Rather, there may be an interim set of conditions that must be established first in order for food to affect behavior, at least in a dramatic way, such as in the case of ADHD. That interim set of conditions may well start with insulin resistance and its partner in crime, inflammation.

Inflammation and the brain

"There is emerging evidence that insulin resistance triggers an inflammatory response in the central nervous system that, in turn, activates unique kinase pathways in neurons," said Jeffrey Bland, PhD, scientist, bestselling author, and founder of the Personalized Lifestyle Medicine Institute in Seattle, Washington. Dr. Bland is one of the world's leading experts on insulin and insulin signaling. "That means that anything that causes inflammation in the central nervous system, including excess sugar consumption, or a sedentary lifestyle, or exposure to toxic heavy elements, can alter the inflammatory pathways, cause insulin resistance, and trigger kinase alterations," said Dr. Bland.

Those changes in kinase patterns can indeed change the way the brain functions, which in turn can alter perception and behavior.

Several food substances lead to insulin resistance and inflammation, especially processed foods, sugar, and saturated fat—the very foods Feingold and others have identified as the causes of ADHD. Dr. Bland takes the theory even further.

"All agents that the central nervous system perceives as 'foreign' might initiate an inflammatory response which in turn modifies kinase signaling, insulin sensitivity, and insulin signaling," he said.

Clearly artificial colors, flavors, and preservatives are foreign to human biology, especially when you consider that they have only come into widespread use during the past 40 years. The same might be said about the quantities of sugar and processed foods that we are eating today.

Some children are biologically more sensitive

Although these substances are foreign to all of us, it's very possible that some children are genetically designed to be more sensitive to these substances than others. These sensitive children may be more vulnerable to insulin resistance and inflammation, which might make such conditions more acute, and thus result in more severe symptoms—including ADHD.

The relationship among food, lifestyle, and brain dysfunction is gaining increasing support from our growing understanding of signal transduction, which is revealing the underlying biology for how things go awry when insulin function is thrown off.

Insulin resistance as one possible theory

Scientists are finding that insulin resistance can spread from the body cells to the cells of the central nervous system and the brain. Once there, they can have a profound effect on brain function, causing, among other conditions, dramatic changes in brain formation and psychological health.

Once insulin resistance takes hold in the brain, it can alter the delicate communication that occurs within neurons and between them, causing dramatic changes in brain function and altering perceptions, thoughts, impulses, moods, and beliefs.

Though still controversial, the theory that insulin resistance is at the bottom of many brain and psychiatric disorders is now finding its way into the some levels of the medical literature. In an article for the *Journal of the American Medical Association* (October 11, 2006), M. J. Friedrich wrote the following:

"Known best for its role in the body as a regulator of blood glucose levels and fatty acid storage, insulin also acts in the brain to aid memory and thinking. Thus, when insulin regulation is disrupted, as it is in many common medical conditions including obesity and diabetes, the risk for cognitive impairment rises."

That cognitive impairment can take many forms—from Alzheimer's disease to ADHD to schizophrenia and bipolar disorder. Certainly there are unique genetic factors that make one person susceptible to, say, ADHD, and another to schizophrenia, and still another to autism. However, increasingly scientists are recognizing that insulin resistance can affect different parts of the brain, and thereby alter gene function, which in turn can trigger one or another of these disorders.

Up until a short while ago, these illnesses were inscrutable to researchers and medical doctors alike. But the new evidence holds out the hope that these seemingly disparate illnesses may one day be treated at their common root. Perhaps even more importantly, researchers are forming the basis for new methods of prevention. Indeed, these approaches may soon give doctors and parents the practical medical and lifestyle tools to control insulin resistance and thereby protect children from these terrible diseases.

The Brain and Glucose: Racing toward burnout

The brain is a high-performance engine. Constantly monitoring every internal system and environmental event, the brain receives billions of bits of information during every instant, organizes the mass of data, and, in most cases, comes up with precisely the right response for the given condition or situation. It is a feat of computer engineering that may never be fully understood, much less matched by human invention.

All that activity, of course, requires energy—lots of it. In fact, your brain requires more glucose and oxygen than any other organ in your body—more than, say, your legs that carry you through each day, or your arms when you are lifting a heavy object. In order for the brain to utilize the available glucose, it must have insulin. But energy delivery is only one of insulin's important tasks. It also regulates how neurons function, which means it plays a key role in how you experience life.

Insulin increases a kinase enzyme known as AKT, which in turn decreases another enzyme, GSK3. The seesaw of those two kinases—as one goes up; the other goes down—allows your brain to produce optimal amounts of the chemical neurotransmitter, acetylcholine, which is essential for you to have memory and awareness of your surroundings—in short, cognition.

But acetylcholine is not the only crucial neurotransmitter regulated by insulin. Another is a substance called glutamate, which is responsible for creating states of arousal and excitement. Glutamate makes cells function more rapidly, much like pushing down on the gas pedal of your car and making the engine race. When glutamate is up, your brain functions much more rapidly.

All well and good, but if you've got too much glutamate, you're not going to be able to sit still for very long, or concentrate on anything for more than a few seconds. You've got to calm down in order to concentrate, to learn, to feel safe, and to enjoy the moment. Among its many duties, insulin regulates glutamate.

Unfortunately, when insulin isn't functioning properly in the brain, it creates complex problems that lead to brain dysfunction. Imagine cells that are forced to race all day and night, but at the same time are not given the raw materials they need to function properly. The engine races, but the materials needed for the cells to do their jobs—such as produce enough neurotransmitter for the brain to function properly—would be missing. Under such conditions, cells would race furiously for a time, burn out, and eventually die. You might experience a lot of arousal and then a big crash into depression. That's basically what happens when insulin cannot regulate glutamate properly. Here's how the problem plays out—at least as far as scientists understand it at this point.

The biology of anguish

Insulin controls glutamate by regulating an array of kinases.

In health, insulin increases production of the kinase AKT, which in turn keeps GSK3 from getting too high. If GSK3 gets too high, your brain will produce more glutamate, which means more of the racing engine. In addition, insulin also promotes the production of a growth factor in the brain known as *brain-derived neurotrophic factor* (or BDNF). BDNF actually buffers the toxic effects of glutamate—rather like eating a pastry in order to protect your stomach from the excess acids caused when you drink too much coffee. The effect of BDNF, therefore, is to protect your brain, in large part by protecting brain cells from the racing and burnout effects of glutamate.

BDNF protects brain cells

In the insulin-resistant brain, there's plenty of glucose and insulin in the blood and tissue, but not enough of either enter the cells. As insulin and glucose drop off, BDNF drops. AKT levels also drop, which means GSK3 goes up. That, in turn, drives ups glutamate. Now cells are racing.

Interestingly, BDNF levels are significantly lower in depressed patients and in other psychiatric conditions. And antidepressants are effective based on their ability to raise BDNF. Furthermore, BDNF has been demonstrated to have antidiabetic effects because the protein enhances insulin sensitivity.

All of which means that BDNF protects your brain cells, works against racing and burnout by slowing things down, and thereby protects against depression and other mental disorders. But this crucial protein depends on proper insulin function. Researchers have found that when glucose and insulin metabolism is impaired, BDNF levels drop. That means that one of the brain's primary protectors has been diminished and is in low supply, thus making the brain susceptible to numerous types of mental disorders. The relationship between insulin and BDNF may well be the crucial link between insulin resistance and psychiatric conditions.

So what causes the inflammation?

Whenever there is racing of cells—the consequence of too much glutamate—there are going to be exhaust fumes. In the brain's case, that means lots of oxidation, free radicals, and inflammation. Immune cells arrive in the brain tissue and attempt to clear the free radicals, but whenever immune cells show up in large numbers, they themselves produce inflammatory cytokines, oxidants, and free radicals, all of which can heighten the levels of inflammation in the body, including in the brain.

Dr. Bland points out that that inflammation even further throws off GSK3, which means that you're going to get even higher glutamate levels, greater metabolic activity, heightened arousal, and all of its related side effects.

Keep in mind that both ends of the age spectrum are affected by these imbalances. For the young person, there is much greater risk of ADHD and, for those who are genetically vulnerable, greater possibility of schizophrenia or bipolar disorder. For the elderly person, the elevated inflammation and higher GSK3 means lower acetylcholine, poorer memory, and greater risk of Alzheimer's disease.

While scientists search for answers to ADHD, schizophrenia, bipolar disorder, and even autism, are there any strategies that are within our control?

Researchers are consistently finding that the omega-3 fatty acids in fish oils, flax seed oils, walnuts, canola oil, and olive oil optimize insulin function and have an antidepressant effect.

Researchers led by Dr. Pnina Green of Tel Aviv University recently reported in the *Journal of Lipid Research* (June 2005) that the brains of depressed laboratory animals contain far higher levels of omega-6 fatty acids, especially arachidonic acid, common in corn oil, soy oil, safflower oil, and processed foods.

Conversely, those with optimal brain function had higher levels of omega-3 fatty acids in their brains. Researchers found that although the depressed animals did indeed have omega-3 fatty acids in their brain, the key was in the balance of omega-3 to omega-6.

"The finding that in the depressive rats the omega-3 fatty acid levels were not decreased, but arachidonic acid was substantially increased as compared to controls is somewhat unexpected," the scientists reported. "But the finding lends itself nicely to the theory that increased omega-3 fatty acids intake may shift the balance between the two fatty acids families in the brain."

Researchers Y. Osher and R. Belmaker at Beer Sheva University in Israel demonstrated in the *CNS Neuroscience Therapeutics* (2009) that omega-3 fatty acids were significantly more effective than placebo for depression in both adults and children.

A diet rich in fish and seafood—excellent sources of omega-3 fatty acids and olive oil and low in processed foods (such as the Mediterranean diet) has been demonstrated to enhance mood and brain stamina.

CHAPTER 11

———

Food, Cells, and Genes

We should all be asking ourselves what can we do to protect ourselves as well as our loved ones from multiple illnesses that arise from the breakdown of our systems biology.

The beginning of the book outlined the delicate process upon which human health rests—the passing of vital information within and between cells also known as signal transduction. The illnesses we suffer from today are caused by bad information being passed to cells, which in turn alters the functioning of our genes, with terrible consequences. An effective solution lies in changing the information that our cells and genes receive. As simple as it seems, we can do that by changing the types of food we eat and by exercising daily.

Food affects our genes

For the past 50 years, nutrition science has been dominated by the language of fats, carbohydrates, calories, vitamins, minerals, and fiber. Today, a new understanding of food and its effects on our bodies is emerging. That new science sees food, literally, as packages of information. The food items that we recognize as beef, whole grains, pasta, or vegetables are, from the standpoint of our cells, bunches of code, packages of information. The nutrients and phytochemicals in food serve as commands at the cellular and genetic levels. Those commands regulate gene expression and thus every bodily function.

Scientists are now finding that foods that are created largely in food factories present our bodies with very different types of information than those that are produced by nature. From the standpoint of our cells, that Krispy Kreme doughnut presents a very different set of command codes than, say, a couple of apples.

Things get far more complicated, and thus far more dangerous, when bits of information are introduced into our bodies that are extremely foreign to our biology. We're talking about all those artificial flavors, colors, preservatives, and pesticides that are in our food. These too are tiny packets of information that affect the way our cells and genes function. The problem is that they are giving the wrong messages, signals, and instructions.

"Our food contains all kinds of additives, emulsifiers, and preservatives, and these substances send information to the body that our genes are not used to receiving," said Dr. Bland of the Lifestyle Medicine Institute in Seattle, one of the nation's leading scientists specializing in the study of how food affects human genes.

"The genes that are turned on as a consequence of the foods that we eat today are the genes that might be collectively and symbolically known as those of Mars, the god of war," said Dr. Bland. "The color is red, which is a symbol for inflammation. The signal is alarm. The foods we eat are causing widespread alarm throughout the system." And that alarm is triggering chemical changes throughout the body that lead to disease and premature death.

The primary source of that alarm, of course, is processed foods—foods that have been altered from their original state and had their calories packed and concentrated into smaller and smaller packages. Processed foods, with their calories and their chemicals, have the body seeing red!

Evolution of food consumption

For most of human history, we consumed food essentially in its natural state—in the case of plant foods, directly from the branch, vine, stem, and root; in the case of animal foods, directly from the bones of the animals we killed. These were, indeed, the first "natural foods"—no artificial anything.

Cooking, of course, was the first form of food processing, but even that did not occur during the first 1.5 million years of our evolution. In fact, no one knows for certain when our earliest ancestors started cooking food, but we probably got the idea when game was roasted in a forest fire and one of our curious forebears put the blackened carcass in his mouth. The first of our cave-dwelling relatives to use fire to prepare food was probably *Homo erectus*, who lived some 700,000 years ago, but scientists debate when he might have started barbecuing. It could have come as late as 400,000 years ago.

From there, it took a very long time for the art of food processing to arise. The Egyptians began making bread and beer round 5,000 BCE, some 7,000 years ago. The people of mid and lower Asia—today's Iraq, Iran, and Afghanistan—began making cheese around the same time. About 4,500 years later, at around 2,500 BCE, the Chinese began to process and produce salt, an art that was further refined in India 1,000 years later. Sugar, derived from sugar cane, didn't appear until 500 BCE, again in India.

Every culture has had its own form of food processing. The Chinese, Japanese, and Indonesians brought food processing to a high art with the development of bean products, such as miso, shoyu, tamari, tempeh, and tofu. Many more foods, the world over, were derived from whole grains. For the most part food processing, no matter how creative, was minimal, meaning that the food itself was not significantly altered from its original state. The grain for bread was crushed and sifted a bit, but the bread itself retained much of its fiber and nutrient content; there were no artificial preservatives introduced to improve shelf life, no colors to enhance appearance. The foods were not fortified with synthetically derived nutrients, nor did they lose many nutrients during processing. There were no artificial emulsifiers, nor artificial forms of fat, such as hydrogenated oils and trans fats, which are common in processed foods today.

In a very real sense, the information conveyed in traditionally processed foods was essentially the same as that derived from nature's food. Traditional processing maintained the essential integrity of the food, and therefore the integrity of the information flowing to the body.

That all began to change in United States in the 1950s.

What is the problem with processed food?

There are many forms of processing that are carried out today. But for the most part, processing means taking a large quantity of food, cooking it, removing the fiber and many nutrients, drying it, and concentrating the calories into a smaller volume of food. For example, corn, a relatively low-calorie food, is transformed into corn chips, a high-calorie food. Wheat, another low-calorie food, is used to make rolls and bagels, both much richer in calories.

Very often, food manufacturers add fat to processed foods, which drives up the calorie content even further. Potato chips, cookies, pastries, and muffins are common examples.

In most cases, processing also means introducing synthetically created chemicals in the form of preservatives that will allow a food to keep from decaying—or going bad—while on your grocery store shelf. In addition, many different flavors, colors, and fats are added to enhance taste and appearance.

One of the lessons we are learning from our experience with processed foods is that the more artificial the food, the more foreign—and therefore more harmful—the information flowing to the body. Trans fats are a good example. A study published in the January 2011 issue of the *Journal of Food Science and Technology* (Vandana Dhaka Neelam Gulia, et al.) reported that trans fats significantly increase insulin resistance, inflammation, overweight, and the risk of both diabetes and heart disease. Researchers at the Harvard School of Public Health have found that each 2% increase in trans fats raises a woman's risk of coronary disease by 93%. By comparison, the researchers have found that for every 5% increase in saturated fat, a woman's chances of having heart disease increases 17%.

Then there is the addition of sugar and artificial flavors, all of which are designed to arouse taste buds. In many cases, caffeine and other substances have been added in order to heighten that arousal even further.

Assault on the body

In a very real sense, processed foods assault the body with far too much information. The overabundance of calories, saturated fat, and artificial ingredients is essentially a massive blitz on our cells. That avalanche of information has widespread effects on our biology. Shortly after consuming a meal containing processed foods, we find the blood engorged with too much glucose, too much cholesterol, too many triglycerides, and too many inflammatory cells. All of these factors disrupt insulin signaling and precipitate inflammation throughout the body, including the nervous system and brain.

Excess information is confusing to both our senses and

our cells. A visit to Times Square in Manhattan after dark is exciting, as it provides a heightened sensory experience. You will find yourself overwhelmed by lights, colors, noise, heights, faces, and bodies in motion. Regular visits will certainly make you inured to the explosion of information flowing to your senses.

The modern diet is having a similar effect on our bodies. Like drugs, our food today is manufactured to create peak experiences. The body is instantly ablaze with inflammatory compounds and excitatory hormones and neurotransmitters, all of which change mood and alter our perceptions.

As with all drugs, rapid elevations are followed by precipitous falls. Blood sugar and neurochemistry levels drop, causing declines in energy, mood, and mental function. A wide array of physical and mental disorders is among the consequences of this rollercoaster ride in blood sugar, hormones, and neurotransmitters.

Dramatic health decline

Once these lows set in, the brain triggers cravings for the addictive food substances—whether it's a burger, milkshake, or sugary snack. Nowhere have the addictive and destructive effects of our modern diet been better demonstrated—at least anecdotally—than by Morgan Spurlock's 2003 documentary film, Super Size Me.

Spurlock, who at the time was 33 years old, went on a 30-day diet that consisted entirely of foods sold at McDonalds. Before going on the diet, he underwent extensive medical examinations by three medical doctors, all of whom proclaimed him in excellent health. Those same physicians followed Spurlock closely during his month-long ordeal and documented his steady—not to mention terrifying—decline in health. Blood tests revealed a precipitous rise in cholesterol, triglycerides, and inflammation, as well as an equally dramatic decline in liver function. After Spurlock was on the McDonald's diet for a couple of weeks, one of his doctors told him that his liver functions resembled that of an alcoholic's. If he continued, his doctor warned him, his liver would fail. Meanwhile, Spurlock rapidly gained weight, suggesting that he was becoming increasingly insulin resistant.

In addition to the measurable declines in health, Spurlock also experienced depression and a decline in energy, and mental and sexual function.

Remarkably, even as his health was failing, Spurlock admitted that he found himself craving the McDonald's food, and that he needed more and more of it to cause the same kinds of emotional highs and feelings of well-being that were associated with the food. He was becoming addicted to McDonald's fast food blend of fatty meats, soft buns, sugary soft drinks, and desserts.

The same has been documented by Damon Gameau in *That Sugar Book* and the accompanying documentary, shining a light on the often toxic effects of sugar on the body—even from so called "healthy" sources such as muesli bars, fruit juices, and healthy snacks.

Children throughout the world find themselves in this same dilemma—they're addicted to foods that are causing them to be overweight, they are becoming insulin resis-

KASH, FRIEDLAND, & LOMBARD

tance and prediabetic as well as developing breakdowns in systems biology such as widespread inflammation .

"The conditions we have today—that is, a diet and lifestyle that creates insulin resistance and inflammation—may be the reasons why we are seeing an increase in dementia, brain inflammation, nonalcoholic fatty livers, cardiovascular disease, and many common cancers," said Dr. Bland. "All of these are manifestations of the information molecules that come from a diet that was really manufactured for the purpose of shelf stability, and not for the purpose of nutrition and health."

Chaotic and deadly effects

Therein lies the problem. The economics of convenience, of shelf life, of instant gratification—these are the driving forces that are actually creating our food supply today. Our multiple epidemics testify to their effects.

For two million years, nature determined our food choices. Today, economic forces and food manufacturers determine to a great extent what we eat. With that change have come new, foreign commands to our cells and genes, with chaotic and deadly effects.

"As the population ages, we're going to see even greater numbers of people suffering from these very diseases, which, many economists predict, will have catastrophic effects on our health care system," says Dr. Bland.

Just as processed food overwhelms us with certain kinds of data, they also convey too little of the kinds of information the body depends upon for health.

Scientists have yet to identify and understand all the chemicals in any given plant food. A single stalk of broccoli, for example, is said to contain literally thousands of phytochemicals. It's possible that every one of those substances play an important role in human health.

In fact, according to Dr. Bland, the unprocessed animal and plant foods contain substances that actually regulate every one of our genes and biological functions.

"When you think about the kinds of foods—and hence the kinds of information—on which we evolved, you must consider that the diet was composed of unprocessed proteins and plants, and that such a diet was consumed over many, many millennia," said Dr. Bland. "Over time, a symbiosis developed between our food and the workings of our genes."

Superiority of plant foods

"Plant foods are enormously complex. They contain a rich array of minerals, flavonoids, polyphenols, nucleic acids, tocopherols, and tens of thousands of other phytochemicals. As we ate these foods and evolved, we came to depend on these substances in order to regulate gene expression and sustain health. Rather than create messages from the 'god of war,' these foods send very different messages to our genes. They create signaling processes that regulate insulin sensitivity. They regulate cell division and repair. They determine gastrointestinal function—our ability to absorb nutrients and eliminate waste. They determine the strength and balance of the immune system, and consequently regulate inflammatory responses. All of these functions are harmoniously controlled by eating a diet that is composed of foods that we refer to as minimally processed," explains Dr. Bland.

All of these chemicals—which number in the tens of thousands—cannot be provided by a supplement, or any form of food fortification. The only way these compounds can be obtained is by consuming a wide variety of plant foods and only a very small amount of unprocessed animal proteins. Like many other health experts, Dr. Bland points to the Mediterranean diet as an ideal model. "In the Mediterranean diet, animal protein is not the centerpiece, as it is in the American diet," says Dr. Bland. "Vegetables, beans, and whole grain products are the center of the diet. And everything is minimally processed. And if you look at the health of people who follow such a diet, you see that they have lower rates of the common illnesses than we do on a highly processed, meat-centered diet."

Traditional diets around the world have many similarities in common. The Asian diet, like the Mediterranean, is centered around plant foods and supplemented by animal proteins. So too were many African and South American diets. The foods throughout the traditional world are minimally processed and nutritionally rich. And not surprisingly, the populations who live on them experience low rates of illnesses that are skyrocketing in the US and other modern countries.

Such traditional diets are delicious, satisfying, and easy to adopt. Indeed, they are also the foundation of our health.

Dietary recommendations to reduce inflammation

Researchers are now virtually unanimous in their recommendation that we adopt a diet that is based largely on plant foods. The reasons are many, but here are some of the most important.

1. Plant-derived foods are generally lower in calories. Plant foods, rich in fiber and water, will fill you up and keep your calorie intake down. This may assist you in losing weight, if you are overweight, or keep your weight low, without causing hunger. Examples:

- Unprocessed whole grains, such as brown rice, barley, millet, oats, and quinoa. A 3½-ounce serving of boiled brown rice contains approximately 130 calories. Oatmeal, barley, millet, and quinoa are even lower in calorie content. If you are not on a calorie-restriction diet, you can comfortably eat two servings per day of whole, unprocessed grains. A diet dominated by whole foods—whole grains, vegetables, and fruit—will allow you to be fully sated and at the same time will promote optimal, healthy weight.

- Green and leafy vegetables, such as bok choy, broccoli, Brussels sprouts, spinach, and general vegetables, as we have already emphasized, are low in calories. A pound of broccoli is 130 calories; a pound of cauliflower, 110; a pound of spinach, 100. Eat at least three servings of green and leafy vegetables daily. Serving size doesn't matter. Eat until you are satisfied.

- Squash, tubers, and roots. Like green and leafy vegetables, they are low in calories and rich in nutrition. Eat at least one serving per day of sweet vegetables, such as squash, tubers, or roots.
- Beans. Four servings per week. A pound of lentils or beans is approximately 530 calories.
- Fruit. At least one serving per day.

Contrast these numbers with high-fat animal foods (fried chicken with the skin is 1,190 calories per pound; hot dogs, 1,500 calories per pound) and processed foods (Stouffer's French Bread Pizza, 1098 calories, or Health Valley fat-free whole wheat crackers, 1620 calories.)

As we have already seen, weight loss changes the types of hormones produced by the adipose tissue, especially adiponectin, a substance that protects us against insulin resistance, cardiovascular disease, and various forms of cancer.

2. They are slowly absorbed, keeping insulin levels low. Whole, unprocessed grains, beans, vegetables, and fruit contain long chains of complex carbohydrates that are encased in long strands of fiber. In order for the carbohydrates to be released from the fibrous matrix, they must be worked on by the intestine, a process that takes hours. Gradually, these sugars are dripped into the bloodstream, causing a steady flow of energy to the body. All of which means that these foods are slowly absorbed. They keep glucose and insulin levels low or normal. They lower inflammation and promote insulin sensitivity, weight loss, and cardiovascular health.

3. The simple sugars found in processed foods, on the other hand, are rapidly absorbed into the bloodstream. Some of the sugars in a candy bar, for example, are absorbed into the bloodstream through the tongue. Once in the blood, these simple sugars cause a rapid rise in glucose and insulin levels, which in turn leads to high levels of blood fats, weight gain, and eventually to insulin resistance.

4. They are low in saturated fat and trans fats, which makes them anti-inflammatory. Saturated and trans fats are two of the most inflammatory substances in the food supply, and thus are part of the reason we are suffering from a pandemic of degenerative diseases. Most unprocessed plant foods are extremely low in saturated fat. Moreover, they contain no trans fats (only processed foods contain these types of fats).

5. Plant foods contain good fats. As we saw in chapter 4, plant foods, rich in polyunsaturated and monounsaturated fats, increase production of the hormone leptin, which enhances insulin sensitivity and may promote weight loss.

6. They are rich in phytochemicals that reduce inflammation and prevent disease. Plant foods are the most abundant sources of substances that boost the immune system, protect cells from insult and mutation, lower cholesterol, and improve circulation to cells throughout the body.

In addition, you will want to adopt an exercise program that will help you lose weight and fight inflammation and insulin resistance.

Exercise as protection against disease

Exercise is highly anti-inflammatory. It also dramatically improves insulin sensitivity. You do not have to strain yourself in order to gain the benefits of exercise. A daily, 30–40 minute walk, will lower insulin, burn fat, and inhibit inflammation. If you cannot walk for a full 30–40 minutes, keeping moving by taking the stairs, including shorter walks during the day and walking to nearby meetings will have the same cumulative effects.

The best exercise program, however, is composed of three parts.

1. Cardio activity: Cycling, jogging, swimming and walking are all excellent, at least three times a week. A great idea is to engage in a physical activity that you enjoy two or three times per week. This could be a sport, such as tennis, basketball, racquetball, swimming, canoeing, or kayaking. It could be a martial art, such as Tai Chi, Chi Gong, Karate, or Aikido. Take a yoga class or a course in ballroom dancing, Tango, swing, Flamenco, or aerobic dancing. Or you could work out at your local gym. Caution. Before you take up a competitive sport, ensure you go for a full physical examination with your medical doctor. For those with cardiovascular risk factors, over-exertion can put you at risk, so do check it out with your doctor first.
2. Strength training
3. Flexibility and stretching
4. Be active throughout the day. Walk up stairs

whenever possible. Avoid elevators to the lower floors. Take short brisk walks on errands. Get out of your chair and move your body.

These illnesses challenge us to examine some of our most accepted and cherished behaviors, including our food choices, exercise habits, and the ways we cope with stress. They also demand that we turn a more sophisticated and even skeptical eye at some of the powerful forces that shape our society and encourage us each day to consume more high-fat, high-protein, and highly processed foods—foods that virtually guarantee the kinds of epidemics that are rampant. It is obviously not just diet alone, but the levels of stress in our lives, which encourages us to use food and escapist entertainment as analgesics against the pain of modern life. The sheer ubiquity of escapist entertainment, especially on television and computers, encourages us—and our children—to live ever more sedentary lives. A sedentary lifestyle, especially when it is joined by the modern diet, is a guarantee for elevated insulin, weight gain, high levels of inflammation, and an increased risk of major disease.

We are informed by a convincing body of scientific evidence that the diet we are enticed to eat, and the lifestyle we are thrilled to enjoy, is killing us. And the more we surrender to the current norms in diet and lifestyle, the greater our chances of becoming overweight, diabetic, and suffering any number of serious illnesses, including heart disease and cancer.

Once any of these degenerative diseases manifest, doctors do all they can to treat them. But as we know, there are limits to what medicine can do. Increasingly, truly effective treatment is seen as a partnership between doctor and patient, for the simple reason that there are things the patient can do that the doctor cannot, and those acts of self-healing can make a world of difference.

CHAPTER 12

Your Health Checklist

The behaviors that affect our hormones and biology are so familiar for many of us that we don't think much about them. The common side effects of high glucose and high insulin—weight gain, along with fluctuations in energy and mood—are often viewed as the normal effects of aging, or a temporary phase that we may be going through. All too often, the small warning signs of inflammation or adrenal and hormonal strain are neglected. Gradually, the conditions get worse until the day we realize that something is very wrong and we're suddenly thrown into crisis.

Following is a simple checklist, along with some medical signs and symptoms, that can alert you to the possibility that your glucose and insulin levels may be too high and that it's time to change your behaviors.

The first part of this checklist is a series of questions

that will give you a good, clear picture of the ordinary symptoms that high insulin—and especially insulin resistance—can cause. The questions can serve as an important tool to reflect on your overall health and provide the basis for an informative discussion that you can have with your doctor.

Following the list of questions is information on a series of blood tests that your doctor can administer to determine if you are, indeed, insulin resistant. Once your doctor knows the specifics of your condition, he or she can offer medications and a diet and lifestyle that can bring your insulin back into normal ranges, and in the process restore your health.

Both the questions and the medical tests are provided by Mark Hyman, MD, who is currently the editor-in-chief of *Alternative Therapies in Health and Medicine*, a peer-reviewed medical journal that covers mainstream and alternative approaches to medicine and health care. Dr. Hyman is also a *New York Times* bestselling author. His many books include *The UltraSimple Diet: Kick-Start Your Metabolism and Safely Lose Up to 10 Pounds in 7 Days* and *Ultra Prevention: The 6-Week Plan That Will Make You Healthy for Life*.

Let's begin with the questions. Give yourself one point for each positive answer. If your score totals five or higher, you should consult your physician and, under his or her guidance, make immediate changes in your diet and exercise habits.

Blood sugar problems (insulin resistance)

1. I crave sweets, eat them, and though I get a temporary boost of energy and mood, I later crash.
2. I have a family history of diabetes, hypoglycemia, or alcoholism.
3. I get irritable, anxious, tired, and jittery, or get headaches intermittently throughout the day, but feel better temporarily after meals.
4. I get dizzy when I stand up quickly.
5. I feel shaky two to three hours after a meal.
6. I eat a low-fat diet and can't seem to lose weight.
7. If I miss a meal I feel cranky and irritable, weak, or tired.
8. If I eat a carbohydrate breakfast (muffin, bagel, cereal, pancakes, etc.) I can't seem to control my eating for the rest of the day.
9. Once I start eating sweets or carbohydrates, I can't seem to stop.
10. If I eat fish or meat and vegetables, I feel good, but seem to get sleepy or feel "drugged" after eating a meal full of pasta, bread, potatoes, and dessert.
11. I go for the bread basket at the restaurant.
12. I get heart palpitations after eating sweets.
13. I seem salt sensitive (I tend to retain water).
14. I get panic attacks in the afternoon if I skip breakfast.
15. Without my morning coffee, I can't get going.
16. I am often moody, impatient, or anxious.
17. My memory and concentration are poor.

18. Eating makes me calm.
19. I get tired a few hours after eating.
20. I get night sweats.
21. I am frequently thirsty.
22. I seem to get frequent infections.
23. I am tired most of the time.
24. I have extra weight around the middle.
25. My hair is thin in the places I don't want it to be thin and grows in the places it shouldn't.
26. I have chronic fungal infections (jock itch, vaginal yeast infections, dry scaly patches on my skin).

I have these diseases, as diagnosed by a medical professional:

27. Polycystic ovarian syndrome or infertility
28. High blood pressure
29. Heart disease
30. Diabetes (adult onset)
31. Cognitive decline
32. Cancer

My blood tests are:

33. Low HDL levels (<50 for men, <60 for women)
34. High triglycerides (>100)
35. Triglyceride/HDL ratio greater than five
36. Abnormal liver function tests or fatty liver
37. High serum ferritin (>200)

38. High serum uric acid (>7.0)
39. Low serum magnesium (<2.0)
40. Fasting blood sugar >90
41. Fasting insulin >8

My sugar intake is:

42. Excessive—I crave and have sweets daily, and drink more than two sweetened or artificially sweetened drinks a day, and eat foods with high fructose corn syrup (food bars, processed food, and so on).
43. High—I eat my share of sugar and sweet foods and crave them, and feel like it is constant struggle to cut down.
44. Moderate—I treat myself occasionally to sweets zero to three times a week.
45. Low—I don't crave or want sugars and eat them very infrequently.

In choosing carbohydrates in my diet, I generally pick:

46. Whole grains like brown rice, quinoa, whole wheat, 100% rye, sweet potatoes, squashes, or whole grain breads or pastas
47. White food—white bread, white rice, bagels, pasta, white potatoes, popcorn, common breakfast cereals

Basic testing for blood sugar imbalance

If, after taking the test, you feel that it would be wise to see your physician, the following tests are among those he or she will want to do to determine if your glucose and insulin levels are excessive, and if you are insulin resistant.

Lipid profile: Blood cholesterol and triglycerides

Your total blood cholesterol should be less than 180 milligrams per deciliter of blood (written as 180 mg/dl).

Your HDL (high density lipoprotein), also known as the good cholesterol, should be greater than 60 mg/dl.

Your triglycerides should be less than 100 mg/dl.

Fasting glucose and insulin tests, accompanied by one-hour and two-hour post-fasting tests

Your fasting glucose should be less than 90.

Your fasting insulin level should be less than 5.

Your one-hour and two-hour insulin level should less than 25.

Your one-hour and two-hour glucose should be less than 120.

Hemoglobin

Hemoglobin is the primary component of red blood cells and carries oxygen within the blood. Doctors run tests on specific fractions of the hemoglobin. Have your doctor test your A1C (HbA1C). It should be less than 5.5.

Fibrinogen

Fibrinogen is a clotting protein produced by the liver. If it becomes excessively elevated, it can lead to increased clots and an increased risk of heart attack and stroke. People with insulin resistance often have higher-than-normal fibrinogen, one of the many reasons they are at an increased risk of heart attack and stroke.

Your fibrinogen level should be lower than 300 mg/dl.

Uric acid

Your kidneys filter uric acid from the blood. People who eat diets rich in animal proteins and fats tend to have high uric acid levels, which can damage the kidneys and lead to gout.

Your uric acid level should be lower than 5.0.

High-sensitivity C-reactive protein

C-reactive protein is a test that can determine the general level of inflammation throughout your body. It can predict your risk of heart disease and other serious illnesses.

Your high sensitivity C-reactive protein level should be less than 0.7.

Ferritin

Ferritin is a protein in the body that stores iron. High iron levels are associated with an array of illnesses, including cancer.

Your ferritin level should be less than 200 milligrams per milliliter of blood.

KASH, FRIEDLAND, & LOMBARD

Liver function tests

High glucose, high insulin, and metabolic syndrome are all associated with decreased liver function. Your doctor may want to run a series of liver function tests on you, including those known by the following ALT, AST, GGT. All three should be within normal limits.

Homocysteine

Homocysteine is an amino acid that rises when we consume excess levels of animal protein. It combines with LDL cholesterol to form a highly inflammatory compound that increases the risk of heart disease.

Your homocysteine levels should be less than 8 mg/dl.

Testosterone levels in men

Male testosterone levels should be greater than 500 mg/dl.

Free-floating testosterone should be greater than 60 mg/dl.

DHEA-S levels in women

DHEA-S (Dehydroepiandrosterone-sulfate) is an important steroid hormone produced in the body and is further converted to testosterone in men and estrogen in women. Women with elevated levels of DHEA-S often suffer from adrenal exhaustion and polycystic ovaries. DHEA-S should be within normal limits (ranges vary depending on the laboratory).

The questions and tests provided here can tell you if you are at risk of having high insulin and even insulin resistance. Only your doctor can confirm your suspicions. That's why we recommend that if you have any of the symptoms described in the questionnaire, you should make an appointment to see your physician as soon as possible.

Acknowledgements

First and foremost, I want to thank my co-authors Dr. Linda Friedland and Dr. Jay Lombard who share my vision on helping end disease through health consciousness and science education. I want to also thank Tom Monte who in our first edition was a guide to the book and more importantly life itself. Our gratitude extends to our agents Jim Levine and Kerry Sparks at Levine Greenberg Rostan Literary Agency and to Lia Ottaviano and Eliza Kirby at Diversion Books who besides publishing books utilize this incredible medium to make a positive change in our beautiful dynamic world. We also give a special thanks to Dr. Mehmet Oz for his words of vision and for all that he does in educating millions about healthcare for themselves and those they love. After witnessing both the suffering and the strength of my mother Leona Kash during her bout with type II diabetes; may this book help to promote a better understanding of the science that will lead us all to a healthy lifestyle. I want to thank my wife and best friend, Donna, who still encourages me to reach new heights, and our four children Jared, Colby, Shantal, and Zena, who make it all worthwhile. I hope that this book helps their generation lead healthier, happier lives. Of course I need to acknowledge my in-laws Marilyn and Herman Freidman, today in their 80s, who practiced healthy eating decades before it was in vogue, and lastly my 90-year-old dad, Robert Kash, from truly the greatest generation.

—Dr. Peter M. Kash

Thank you to my co-authors Peter Kash and Jay Lombard. Peter, much appreciation for the opportunity to partner with you on this project and for opening the doors to so many others. Thank you to Kerry Sparks at Levine Greenberg Rostan Literary Agency and to Lia Ottaviano and Eliza Kirby at Diversion Books and to Dr. Mehmet Oz for the insightful foreword. Gratitude always to my husband Peter Friedland and our children Gavi & Lee, Yael & David, Leora, Aharon, Benjamin and of course Zachary & Samuel.

—Dr. Linda Friedland

I would like to thank my coauthors Linda and Peter for making this edition a reality. Also without our editor, publisher and agent we couldn't help all those in need. A special thanks to our friend Dr. Mehmet Oz for a foreword that truly highlights the message of the book. Most importantly my family for the endless hours they have put up with me when researching nutrition and the brain. Thank you Rita, Julia and Sofia.

—Dr. Jay Lombard